BREAK OUT
OF THE SUGAR PRISON

Copyright © 2009 by Shelly Young and Paul Harris

ISBN: 0-9776128-6-4

    All rights reserved. This book contains material protected under international and federal copyright law and treaties. Any unauthorized reprint, distribution or use of this material is prohibited.

    No part of this publication may be reproduced, stored in a retrieval system or transmitted, in any form or by any means, electronic, mechanical, photocopying, recording, facsimile or otherwise, without the prior written consent of the copyright owners.

Publisher's Note

The health related information and mindfulness practices and suggestions contained in this book are based on the extensive training, research, clinical experience and opinions of the authors. Nothing herein should be misinterpreted as actual medical advice, advice for self-diagnosis or self-treatment. Neither are they to be considered a particular or general cure for any ailment, disease or other physical, emotional or mental health issue.

Because there is always some risk involved in any health-related program, the authors and publisher assume no responsibility for any adverse effects or consequences resulting from the use of any suggested preparations, practices, exercises, formulations or procedures described in this book.

The authors and publisher do not warrant the performance, effectiveness or applicability of any web logs or any other websites which may be listed or mentioned in this book. Any links which may appear in this book are for information purposes only and are not warranted for content, accuracy or any other implied or explicit purpose.

This book is compassionately dedicated to our patients, clients and readers who have demonstrated the willingness to learn what it takes to truly understand and come to grips with the serious nature of sugar addiction and to do something constructive about it.

Acknowledgements

To everyone who helped make this book possible, please know that we sincerely appreciate your timely contributions. Many offered sage advice regarding the technical aspects of text composition and cover design. Others afforded a level of moral support that helped us create and foster the kind of intellectual and spiritual atmosphere necessary to carry out a project of this magnitude.

A special thanks to Shinzen Young, Barbara Harris, Roger Carpenter, Allison St. Claire and Elizabeth Reninger - all of whom so graciously gave of their time and expertise in the careful preparation of this book.

What This Book is About

Have you ever suspected that you might be a "sugar addict?" Do you have tendencies toward consuming sugar in ways that are harmful to you, or perhaps even downright abusive? Do you ever feel out of control with sugar cravings, or notice that you oftentimes eat more than you want to? Do you ever consume cakes, candies, soft drinks, ice cream, processed cereal or other sugar-rich foods until you feel sick? Do you want to stop, but feel that you cannot – as though some mysterious force is compelling you to continue? Do you use sugar to get "high" or to numb yourself out?

Maybe you can't remember a time when sugar bingeing was not part of your life. It may even feel like a "sugar prison." You may have tried to break out, repeatedly, but have not succeeded. You may feel frustrated, hopeless, anxious or depressed about your situation. Perhaps others judge you. Perhaps you judge yourself, with thoughts like: "I have no will power. How could I let myself gain so much weight? I am so stupid for doing this to myself." Maybe you experience feelings of shame and loathing in relation to your body. You may even crave a genuine sense of gratification or "sweetness" in your life, yet somehow have become trapped in something that is not at all satisfying.

In this book you will learn the truth about your sugar addiction. You will come to see that it is not a personal weakness. You will learn the facts about the mind/body components of what you are currently experiencing as your "prison." You will become clear about what the problem really is. You will find solutions within a unique mindfulness approach, with powerful awareness techniques that can help you regain control of your life, and enjoy once again an authentic freedom of choice, moment by moment. You will also learn how to properly care for your body in a way that is completely natural and biologically friendly.

What sets this book apart from many other well-meaning efforts to offer support in turning back the strong tide of sugar addiction is its unique perspective. We view addictive tendencies and the means by which they can be successfully eradicated in a new and integrated way – whose main components are personal initiative, focused and directed mind-body practices, and intelligent nutritional support.

In Part One, certified nutritionist, Paul Harris, former student of the late Dr. Bernard Jensen, explores the effects of sugar on your body in both its constructive and destructive aspects. You will learn how the harmless desire for sugar and sugar byproducts can grow into a hideous monstrosity, capable of controlling every aspect of your life. You will discover how and why this can happen quickly and unexpectedly, and what you can do to unwind these patterns, and regain control of your life-choices.

In Part Two, licensed professional counselor and certified addiction counselor, Shelly Young, presents the mindfulness component of the program. With the support of simple, powerful mind-body awareness techniques, you will quickly discover that your cravings do not have to control your behavior and cause you to engage in self-destructive habit patterns. You will learn body-mind empowerment exercises that will lessen the intensity of cravings, or eliminate them entirely. Shelly will explain how through practicing these simple methods, sugar addiction will cease to have a hold on you, and you can regain a sense of spacious freedom and delight in your life-journey.

The mindfulness methods presented in this book are the brilliant creation of Shinzen Young, author of *Break Through Pain: a Step by Step Mindfulness Meditation Program for Transforming Chronic and Acute Pain*. Shinzen is a well-known and respected senior mindfulness teacher, who leads retreats in the United States and Canada, as well as abroad. He has 40 years of mindfulness practice behind him, and received an honorary Doctorate in 2005 from the Institute for Transpersonal Psychology in Palo Alto, California. Shinzen has authored numerous articles and CD's on various topics relating to his unique teachings. He has spent a

WHAT THIS BOOK IS ABOUT

good portion of his life developing methods that can benefit individuals from all walks of life.

In Part Three you will be introduced to a proven, effective and personally compatible nutritional system - The Sugar Prison Diet - that can support you in quickly reversing the physiological dependency you have on sugar.

In the Appendix you will find many useful aids, such as the *Weekly Diet and Nutrition Worksheets* and the *Daily Mindfulness for Life Worksheet*. You will also find many delicious and healthy recipes, all of which can help you intelligently and enthusiastically overcome your addiction to sugar.

Break Out of the Sugar Prison is a unique endeavor. It represents the first ever combining of powerful Basic States mindfulness techniques with an effective nutritional system. The possibilities of multi-level healing and meaningful discovery that await you are endless.

By the time you finish reading this book, you will have at your fingertips a complete, easy-to-follow and enjoyable, health-restoring protocol. It is a program that can take you from wherever you are now mentally, emotionally and physically, and usher you onward to a wonderful state of whole-being health and wellness. You can come to a place where the dreaded specter of sugar addiction can never again threaten the security and sanctity of your life in any measurable way.

Contents

Acknowledgments — vii
What This Book is About — ix
Preface — ixx
Foreword — xxv
Introduction — xxvii

PART ONE
Introducing the Dragon of Sugar Addiction

Chapter 1: Birth of the Dragon of Sugar Addiction – Your Jailer and Prison Guard — 3
    The Addiction Seed is Planted Early — 4
    Feeding the Dragon Day In and Day Out — 6
    The Hidden How and Why of Sugar-Related Mood Swings — 8
    Should Refined Sugar be Classified as a Drug? — 10
        Not-so-sweet Criminals — 10
        Sugar Bingeing Rats — 11

Chapter 2: More Sugar Woes and Lows — 13
    The Dangerous Affinity of Sugar to Calcium — 13
    Soft Drinks and Sugar Substitutes — 14
    The Case of the Dissolving Tooth — 17

Chapter 3: Getting Your Motor Running — 19
    A Simple and Effective Dietary Program to Help You Reverse Your Sugar Addiction — 19
    Starting Sensibly — 20

PART TWO
Mindfulness: The Basic States System

Chapter 4: Mindfulness: Break Through Your Sugar Addiction and More! — 23

Chapter 5: What is Suffering? — 25
- Hatred — 25
- Clinging — 25
- Unconsciousness — 26

Chapter 6: Lightening the Weight — 29
- Divide and Conquer — 29

Chapter 7: The Basics of Mindfulness Practice — 31
- Concentration, Clarity and Equanimity — 31

Chapter 8: The Significance of Change — 33
- Mindfulness and Nature — 33

Chapter 9: Becoming Aware of the Ordinary — 35
- The Basic Mind/Body States — 35
- Labeling (naming) — 35
- Research — 38

Chapter 10: The Power of Restful States — 41
- Restful States — 41

Chapter 11: Guided Mindfulness Exercises — 43
- Focus In — 43
  - Technique #1: Focus on Image Space — 43
  - Technique #2: Focus on Talk Space — 44
  - Technique #3: Focus on Feel Space — 45
- Focus on Rest — 46
  - Technique #4: Focus on Blank — 46
  - Technique #5: Focus on Relaxation — 46

Focus Out	47
Technique #6: Focus on Touch, Sight, Sound	47

Chapter 12: Getting the Most Out of Mindfulness – The Basic States Method   49
    Sitting Practice   49
    Practice in Action   49

Chapter 13: Abstaining from Sugar Bingeing   51
    Practicing Mindfulness with Sugar Cravings   52

Chapter 14: Eating as a Meditation   53
    Working Through Compulsion and Elevating Satisfaction: Article by Shinzen Young   53

Chapter 15: Mindfulness to Combat Other Destructive Urges   57
    Using Mindfulness Practice to Deal with Negative Urges: Article by Shinzen Young   57

Chapter 16: Shelly's Personal Journey   61
    June 1985 Interview   62
        67

Chapter 17: Cognitive Behavioral Therapy
    Taking an Eclectic Approach to Your Healing   67

Chapter 18: Frequently Asked Questions about the Techniques   71

PART THREE
Learning to Feed Your Body Instead of Your Addiction

Chapter 19: The Sugar Prison Diet   77
    Getting the Best Results from a Therapeutic Fast or 21-Day Transitional Dit   78

Chapter 20: Letting Nature Cleanse, Rest and Rejuvenate Your Body   81

    Step One / Option A – The Powerful Secret of Why a Fast Can Help You Quickly Overcome Your Sugar Addiction   81

    Basic Elements of the Therapeutic Fast   83

    Step-By-Step Guide for Conducting and Finishing the 7-Day Therapeutic Fast   84

    The Proper Way to Break Your Fast   85

    Step One/Option B – 21-Day Transitional Diet   86

    21-Day Menu   87

Chapter 21: Wholesome and Healthy Maintenance Menus   93

    Step Two/Option A – A 30-Day Sample Menu to Use after You Break Your Fast or Complete the 21-Day Transitional Diet   93

    30-Day Sample Menu   95

    Step Two/Option B – Quick and Simple Daily Menu for Busy Sugar Addicts   100

    Healthy Food Items You can Consume after the Fast or 21-Day Transitional Diet   102

    Stay Away from or Minimize Your Use of These Denatured Foods and Beverages   104

    Basic Laws of Eating   105

Chapter 22: Start NOW to Break Out of the Sugar Prison   107

Conclusion   109

Appendix

    Worksheets   113

        Daily Mindfulness for Life Worksheet   114

        Weekly Diet and Nutrition Worksheets   115

    Healthy Recipes 123
        Broth Recipes 124
        Soup Recipes 129
        Protein Recipes 135
        Baked and Cooked Vegetables 143
        Sandwiches 147
        Fruit and Vegetable Cocktails 149
        Nut and Seed Milks 152
        Raw Vegetable Salads 154
    Silicon Tonic 156
    Whole Foods Blended Cocktail 157

References 159

Mindfulness Daily Practice Flash Cards 163

To Contact the Authors 173
About the Authors 175

Preface

Shelly Young: Once upon a time, I walked up and down the colorful streets of Berkeley, California. It was Telegraph Avenue that attracted me most of all. The atmosphere was so bizarre that I was easily distracted from the agonizing feelings of self-loathing, self-pity, hopelessness, fear and despair. There, on Telegraph Avenue, I could forget my swollen ankles, hands and legs - swollen from the consumption of massive amounts of sugary foods and refined carbohydrates. In Berkeley I could lose myself within unusual forms of creative expressions, some of which seemed pathological. You have to know the Telegraph Avenue of the '70s to understand what I mean. I spent day after day, hour upon hour, utterly consumed, obsessed, and tormented by a sugar and food obsession. Sugar was my complete ruination.

Before the Berkeley era, I had abstained from bingeing for seven months while attending Overeaters Anonymous meetings. After relocating to California I fell off the wagon once again and gained fifty pounds in three months. Clinical depression accompanied the bingeing as I approached a non-functional existence. I went to a psychiatrist and was diagnosed with a mood disorder but refused medication. I awoke one morning and groggily opened my change purse only to find one penny. That was a most memorable morning! It was welfare or a psych hospital. I chose welfare and could barely get myself to the office. Along with the welfare came food stamps, a month's worth binged away in three days. I had been accepted into an addiction treatment program but got cold feet at the last minute.

Luckily I could sing well and also played guitar. I phoned a café and got hired but the money was binged away immediately. If I was lucky enough to stop eating I would start chewing. Transformed into a sorbitol junkie, I chewed 20 to 30 packs of sugarless gum per day, chewing gum wrappers strewn all over my room, incessant bouts of daily diarrhea. Berkeley was the place I walked aimlessly every day, trying to make the most out of a quarter.

In 1980 I desperately searched the Bay Guardian, a small San Francisco newspaper, longing for an answer to my living Hell. I saw an advertisement for mindfulness and phoned the teacher immediately. When he answered the phone I asked, "Do you have peace of mind?" He said "yes" in a way that was truly genuine. I made an appointment and was on his doorstep the next day. As he opened the door I could sense a true peacefulness about him. I had met lots of people in my life that smiled a lot, were energetic, charismatic, vivacious and friendly. But I had never met anyone with what I considered to be true peace of mind. I wanted what he had and knew that I would do anything for it. It was on February 24, 1980 - my 29th birthday - that my mindfulness journey began.

I have spent years assisting clients and students in transforming their lives using simple mindfulness techniques. I have witnessed seemingly hopeless individuals attain peace and freedom in the midst of significant personal challenges. Since I am one of those people, I can share my experience and hope for anyone who is seeking relief from the inevitable sufferings of life. My work as a mindfulness-based psychotherapist stems not only from my personal transformation but also a deep belief in every person's ability to discover their own inherent place of internal peace and harmony.

With the assistance of my colleague, Paul Harris, I will explain how *you* can break out of the sugar prison.

Shelly Young
Boulder, Colorado
2009

Paul Harris: When I was a youngster in Queens, New York, my usual habit was to take a candy bar, soft drink, miniature lemon or cherry pie, cookies or some other processed, sugar-rich concoction with me whenever I left the house. It did not matter if I was going to school, to town with one or both of my parents, to the local playground or anywhere else my young, wiry, sugar-craving body desired to go. Sugary snacks had become such a part of my life that I could not imagine going through a day without them.

This habit contributed toward my unhealthy little body becoming host to a number of dreadful, acidic ailments that persisted throughout most of my childhood. Unfortunately for me, my parents were not well-schooled in the fine arts of wholesome meal preparation or holistic health care practice. Their answer to my incessant complaints about nervous tics, upset tummy, gas, painful joints and muscle spasms was to have a local family doctor in Queens, N.Y., inject my young body with every new and virtually untested drug he could conjure.

The result of this drug therapy, coupled with my continued sugar bingeing excesses, was the development of a serious health condition that eventually affected both inner ears. In fact, so serious were these complications that, during the late 1970s through the early '80s, I had to undergo a series of inner ear operations to bring lasting and welcome relief. Following those painful intrusions into my head, I resolved that I would never again subject myself to that kind of pain, distress and discomfort.

Not long after my final ear operation, my mother was diagnosed with a particularly aggressive form of breast cancer. This was the culminating result of many years of smoking and dietary abuse - with a particular focus on excessive sugar consumption. Previous to the diagnosis, she had been a diabetic for most of her adult life. It seemed the grim reaper had his watchful eye on Mom for quite some years and had no intention of lifting his claim on her.

Nothing slowed or diverted the onslaught of her demise. Every bodily system had been adversely affected in structure and function. At a certain point, Mom's oncologist informed my father he could do nothing further for her. Dad drove her up to a Canadian physician who thought his methodologies could help revive her ailing body. This was ill-advised, far too late and, ultimately, to no avail. Within two weeks Mom's kidneys failed and she asked to be returned to New York where she could die at home with dignity amidst friends and family.

This never happened. Instead of going home, Mom was rushed instead to a local hospital in Queens for emergency care. I visited her there. Surrounding her bed, in her stark, private room were my father, brother and his wife, my wife Barbara and myself. A respirator controlled the ebb and flow of Mom's breathing – her life. She had been drugged mercilessly and, consequently was barely coherent.

Curiously, thoughts of my joyful childhood years with Mom filled my mind. She had lived a life to be envied. World traveled; a wonderfully gifted teacher beloved by her many students and their grateful parents; a caring and loving mother to her two sons, and a faithful wife to her hard-working husband. The hallmark of her presence at any social gathering was her crisp and infectious laughter that could fill a large room just as surely and completely as it filled my mind in that hospital room.

These fond memories hovered in stark contrast to the pitiful sight of the ailing, insensible woman who lay before me in submissive repose.

While the others in the room were discussing something among themselves, I sat on the bed at Mom's right side, leaned forward, kissed her sweaty forehead and whispered the following words in her ear:

"I swear to you I will *never* let this happen to anyone else if I can help it."

Mom made no attempt at verbal acknowledgment but slowly, almost imperceptibly, nodded her head so as to let me know she heard and felt what I was saying to her. Tears welled up in my eyes for the first time in years. Waves of anger and sadness rolled through and saturated my being. What happened? How did it happen so quickly? Why didn't anyone in the immediate family inform me about the seriousness of Mom's condition back when I could have stepped in and perhaps turned the tide? These questions kept rumbling in my head like dark storm clouds. Had I known, early on, about the grave condition of Mom's illness I certainly could have made a difference. This story could have had

PREFACE

a cheerful outcome. But this was not the case. I was kept in the dark and rendered ineffectual when it mattered most.

We eventually left Mom alone, in her cold hospital bed, in that bleak room, and went back to my parent's house in Queens. The promise I made to my mother were the last words I ever spoke to her. She passed away a few days after that.

Mom and Dad raised my brother and me to be mentally strong and resilient in the face of all adversity. But this was something I was not prepared for – the sudden and final removal of Mom from my life. It was a painful tearing away of a large piece of my heart and my life. Oh, if I had only taken time from all of my carefree frolicking as a child, thrill seeking adventures as a teenager and stubborn bullheadedness as an adult, and gotten to know her better. Perhaps then I could have earned her trust in my judgment, at a deeper level. Maybe then she would have given heed to my weekly railings against her poor dietary habits and endless cigarette smoking.

Back at my parent's house, the once cheerful, soft orange walls of the second floor den, Mom's favorite room that she had once painted during one of her many inspired moods of artistic creativity, seemed dark, cold, sullen and not so inviting as they were when she graced the room. In fact, the entire house felt as though a heavy, woolen blanket had been laid over it. We were all spell-bound by the finality of what was happening. Mom was the cohesive mortar that had always kept the structure of our family together and now it was rapidly disintegrating. We would have only our cherished memories of Mom to hold onto.

Dad was another person then. He seemed removed, distant and completely unattached to things worldly. Not at all like the outgoing, self assured and confident all American basketball star and league MVP that he was while attending Morehouse College. Nor did he have the lift in his stride and keen optimism he once exhibited while directing special programs for disadvantaged children at school district 15 in Lawrence, Long Island. This was a different man - shocked, hurt and wary about an uncertain future without the love of his life by his side.

I cannot recall how many attempts I made to apologize to my father and brother for not monitoring Mom's health issues more closely over the years. It was a painful experience requiring an enormous surge of courage to face either of them about how and why I missed all of the telltale signs of the impending danger that loomed on the horizon for Mom when it mattered most and may have saved her life. After all, I was the family witch doctor – or so they sometimes jokingly referred to me as. It was my job to ensure everyone in the family could and would benefit from the fruits of my learning.

I thought about how I would cringe at the sight of Mom eating a large slice of chocolate cake when my wife and I would periodically drop by to visit and how she could go through half a box of chocolate covered candies while watching her favorite television programs. I was concerned about it then but never imagined she would allow her craving for all of those decadent sweets to eventually get the best of her. I also thought about the deathbed promise I made to Mom and what it really meant. I didn't know then how I would keep my word to her, but I knew that, somehow, I *would* keep it.

If you should ask what my real motivation may have been behind writing this book with Shelly, please know that I am doing this to fulfill a *solemn promise* I made to my mother while she lay wasting away on her deathbed. When I learned of my mother's condition, it was already too late to make a difference. It was far too late to save her life. I have written this book with Shelly because what we have to share with you *can* make a difference. It can save a life – perhaps your own or the life of someone you live with, work with, socialize with, love or otherwise hold dear.

Paul Harris
Hesperus, Colorado
2009

Foreword

A deep healing of any disorder (particularly an addiction) will often require a complete involvement of all facets of our being and levels of conscious awareness. The merging of the two disciplines presented in this book - mindfulness and cutting-edge nutrition - affords the reader a "frosty" and engaging view of the driving forces behind addictive tendencies from various psychological, emotional and physiological vantage points.

Having read the material presented in this book, it's not hard to imagine that some readers will be motivated and empowered to experience a true spiritual transformation. A complete, 180-degree turning about in the seat of consciousness, that can bestow a sense of utter peace and knowingness about the importance of being in and with the moment at hand in all that we experience. It is from within the rubble of such a rare, earth-shaking revelation that the naturally intuitive mind arises and sees clearly the cause and the remedy for addictive habits.

Ultimately, addiction comes from our inability to experience ourselves completely. Most people experience complete pleasure only occasionally, if ever. Hence their experience of pleasure usually fails to satisfy and turns into "drivenness." Also, most people experience complete pain only occasionally, if ever. Hence, painful urges turn into suffering which they seek to relieve by acting on that urge.

That's the bad news. The good news is that it's possible to train one's consciousness in core attention skills: concentration power, sensory clarity and inward equanimity. These skills, known collectively as mindful awareness, allow you to have a complete experience of pleasure and therefore find fulfillment and be free of compulsion. They also allow you to have a complete experience of uncomfortable urges. By breaking an urge down into its components - mental images, internal talk, physical body sensation and emotional body sensation - you can divide and conquer it. The urge dissolves into a flow of energy and loses its power to control your behavior. The mindfulness exercises presented in this book will show you step by step, how to develop the focusing skills you need to see through both the carrots (pleasant body-mind states) and the sticks (unpleasant body-mind states) that drive human behavior.

Although this book centers around the issue of sugar addiction, the paradigm of mindfulness presented here is immediately applicable to any type or level of drivenness - from the pathological eating disorders suffered by only a few, to the subtle tensions of daily life suffered by almost all.

Shinzen Young

Introduction

Since the Age of Exploration, traders and explorers of good and ill repute have traveled the world in search of new and profitable sources of sugar, one of the most prized culinary ingredients throughout the ages. That was due to the fact that sugar, in its pure, unadulterated state, was once considered to be a reliable and delicious source of minerals and other nutrients, well-suited for the human body. Alas, that was yesteryear.

The harrowing reality of today is that what we call "pure sugar" is most often a refined, denatured imitation of the real, natural item. Our modern-day chemists and food scientists have compromised the chemical structure and taste of natural sugar to the point where most of us actually prefer the processed sweeteners and sugar substitutes to honest-to-goodness, real, organic sugar you find with sugar cane, dates, raw honey, raw fruit and berries. It appears this trend will continue well into the future.

There are two sides to the sugar story. Sugar is *not* a thing to be feared and completely avoided. In fact, if you neglect to consume foods which can eventually break down into some form of sugar your body can use for heat and energy, you will put yourself in a dangerous and precarious position with regard to your overall health and wellness. You *must* eat carbohydrates and make sugar available to your blood and cells.

The trick, as with everything in nature, is to find a sensible level of balance. On the one hand, you want to ensure efficient, ongoing physiological function and mental and emotional equilibrium. This requires the steady consumption, digestion and assimilation of many essential nutrients, one of which is sugar. On the other hand, you must ensure your intake of sugar, and foods that break down into simple sugar, is not excessive. For quite a number of us, this can be a difficult thing to do. But do it you must if you wish to be well, whole, and vibrantly healthy in mind and body.

There is an inherent or built-in uncertainty about what we think we know regarding sugar and nutritional science in general. That can be partly attributed to the fact that the more we learn about sugar, the more questions arise that, inevitably, lead to more searching, more discovery and yet more questions. A large percentage of the body of information we call nutritional science is founded on certain commonly accepted assumptions which, in turn, rely on a *lot* of faith and belief. We have today, at our disposal, a large and ungainly mass of not-so-nicely-fitting pieces of nutritional knowledge that are the cherished fruits of many brilliant avenues of holistic theory, yet which often conflict in synergistic, practical application.

Those of us involved in the field of nutritional science research and clinical care are often eager to put forth smart-sounding propositions and theories of how we like to *think* our bodies work along certain natural lines and how our theories should universally apply to similar health issues. As ongoing discoveries in the field prove to us all, with each passing day, sometimes we are right and we hit a grand slam. At other times, well, we can't get to first base.

The average person on the street assumes that our nutritional research trials and findings are reflective of real world scenarios. The fact that so many adults faithfully purchase what they think are safety-net vitamin and mineral preparations each month is proof in the pudding they want to, and usually do, believe that what we in the nutritional field tell them is good for their health is, in fact, true. This requires a large and trusting leap of faith that can be dangerous for anyone suffering with a life-threatening disorder or simply attempting to overcome an addiction to sugar or to any other abused substance.

What the general public rarely suspects is that those of us who are entrusted to provide reliable nutritional information are ever hopeful we are not dispensing information today, to patients and readers, that may prove unsound or downright unsafe for those same patients and readers tomorrow. From our precarious intellectual perch, we observe exciting research findings and new ways of taking care of old ailments. Unfortunately, we must also give audience to occasional, unwelcome stories about adverse reactions to promising nutritional supplements or revolutionary natural therapies.

With all of the smoke and mirrors abounding in the field of health care, it can be quite a task determining what makes sense for you as an individual. Variance in body types, genetic makeup, psychological and emotional factors and efficiency of physiological function, from one person to the next, are some of the factors that can make our job as providers of reliable information applicable to the general public so difficult. There are far too many physical, emotional and mental considerations to take into account to make sweeping generalizations about any supposed failsafe supplements or therapies that can be applied, on a broad scale, or even to you in your personal battle with sugar addiction.

The best of theories about the harmful effects of sugar addiction, and effective approaches to treatment and intelligent psychological consultation to reverse addictive tendencies, can only find justification in their actual working out in the real world. That is the testing ground, the real battlefield we should be paying attention to. It is only then - when the ship of theory has been built in the factory of reasonable proposition and set to sail on its maiden voyage upon the sea of common sense - that any respectable and believable assertions can and should be made about the ship's ability to reach the far shore of nutritional fact and certainty. That is the time to cast in your lot with a winning formula – when you know, with certainty, that those who would chart for you a course to reverse your addictive tendencies to sugar have previously discovered that distant and elusive land for themselves.

Toward that end I can assure you the sugar addiction reversal protocol described in this book is the result of many years of direct patient care and careful research. It has been our earnest desire to separate truth and reality from theory and assumption. All that you will encounter in the protocol has been worked out, *in the real world*, by me and by my colleague, Shelly Young. There is little theory imbedded within the confines of our game plan - with its symbiotic mindfulness and nutrition-driven components. The chances are high that the message we will impart to you, in this book, can be of benefit to you in your quest to overcome your sugar addiction or habitual and excessive consumption of sugar and its many byproducts.

Join us now on a journey to a special place where your earnest effort to regain your health can bring you closer to soundness of mind, body and spirit. Together we will visit nature's inner sanctum where you will learn about her unchanging laws of right eating, right living and right mindfulness. A timeless place where you can reclaim your life and purpose and discover a powerful and effective way to overcome any addictive or abusive tendencies you may have towards sugar or any other food, drink or substance. Come with us to the land of whole-being health and wellness and addiction-free living.

PART ONE

Introducing the Dragon of Sugar Addiction

CHAPTER 1

Birth of the Dragon of Sugar Addiction-Your Jailer and Prison Guard

Your addiction to sugar is like a fire-breathing dragon. It is little more than a demanding jailer - a prison guard - that keeps you locked up inside your own self-erected and self-imposed sugar prison.

If your sugar habit has progressed to the point where you feel physically, emotionally and mentally locked inside the sugar prison, there is a good reason for that. You can bet that if you feel overwhelmed by the sheer magnitude or ferocity of your addiction, there is a large, imposing and perpetually hungry dragon orchestrating your predicament. It relentlessly monitors your every thought, feeling and action to determine how to maximize its absolute control and power over you, your freedom and your life.

As your desire and need for sugar grows, so also does your dragon. It will continue to grow, unabated, until you do something decisive about it. Yet, until that day comes along, your self-imposed sugar prison is steadily under construction all around you. Haven't you noticed that whenever your addictive sugar dragon has sent you in search of tasty sugar snacks, treats or starchy meals, that you have had a heavy, seemingly unbreakable chain tightly bound around your neck? Your dragon - the raw desire fueling your addictive habit - will only let you wander far enough away from the prison each day to find another sweet meal or treat. Then it will quickly haul you back into the prison.

Try as you may to wake up from your nightmare, you feel powerless to undo your horrid circumstances. You feel your situation is desperate and the dragon is well aware of this. In fact, it thrives on your insecurity and paranoia. The dragon knows that if a random, rebellious thought were to ever enter your mind you would quickly dismiss it as a task fit for someone with greater resolve. Your dragon is crafty, clever, bold and supremely confident. It has been growing in size, purpose and, I dare say, arrogance since you gave it life. The key to defeating and subduing the dragon is understanding what it really feeds on every day. It is feeding on your *desire* and *craving* for sugar - nothing more.

Your uncontrolled desire for sugar is what the dragon considers necessary for its survival and well-being. And it knows with dead certainty that as long as your mouth waters and your tummy growls when you contemplate a delicious sweet snack or a meal of starchy carbohydrates, that you will continue to supply its favorite meal – desire, which is its life energy.

The Addiction Seed is Planted Early

Children at play, and during other times of physical exertion, require vast stores of sugar for instantaneous energy conversion. Sugar enables this rapid-fire electrochemical process to take place. Any available blood sugar is called upon for immediate utilization. Whenever the body's energy requirements exceed available blood sugar, the body will quickly convert glycogen stored in muscle tissue and in the liver into glucose, which can be converted into energy. Although stored fatty tissue can be used for this purpose, to some extent, it is sugar in its simplest forms that a child's body prefers for energy conversion.

A child learns early on that the sugar-sweetened bubble gum, candy bars, soda pop, sweet ice cream and milk shakes, and pies and cakes give a quick energy boost. Soon the child identifies energy production and feeling good with processed carbohydrates in their many forms. The earliest roots for sugar addiction begin to grow and take hold during the formative years.

Meanwhile, certain physiological, mental and emotional phenomena are occurring as all of this sugar is pouring in unchecked. At the physical level, the organs and glands responsible for sugar metabolism are hyperactive, working at a breakneck pace to keep up with the need to mitigate the harmful effects of excessive sugar being present in your blood and tissues. The first signs of physical discomfort appear in the form of excess mucous and inflamed and swollen mucus membranes. Typically, parents give the child over-the-counter or prescription drugs to relieve the condition, not knowing the discharge is nature's way of attempting to mitigate the destructive onslaught of sugar abuse.

The symptom-suppressing treatments drive the harmful waste materials back into the body, where they usually settle in weak organs, glands and other compromised tissue. These underperforming, waste-bearing areas become breeding grounds for future pathology. The sugar prison's foundation is under construction.

After a time the organs and glands that have been weakened by their continual hyper- activity start to give in to the pressure. The pancreas and adrenals become erratic in their hormonal output, the pituitary, thyroid and hypothalamus have great difficulty influencing a stable blood sugar level, and the liver is partially incapacitated in controlling sugar metabolism in the body.

As the liver and thyroid are functionally compromised, emotional instability, feelings of insecurity, stress, sadness, depression and paranoia are but a handful of the many complications that can arise as the brain is not fed proper levels of sugar and other needed nutrients. Too little electrical stimuli are sent to the heart, lungs and the organs of elimination.

This steadily decreasing electrical stimulation leads to chronic weakness of the affected organs and glands, inefficient hormonal production, enervation, cellular waste buildup, malnutrition, and overall reduced bodily function and efficiency. If the child's condition is not corrected by natural means, this can eventually lead to a chronic state of affairs where nerve force, vitality and blood flow to affected areas are partially or completely arrested. If this continues into adulthood, serious ailments such as cancer, arthritis, emphysema, nephritis and circulatory disorders, may arise in perfect accord with the rising walls of the sugar prison.

Even in the face of such dire possibilities, our natural tendency is to keep doing whatever it is that makes us feel good until we start feeling bad. Have you been on this wild merry-go-round, thinking the ride and fun would last forever? I know I did. And I suffered because of it for many years.

Feeding the Dragon Day In and Day Out

If you find pleasure in a given experience, such as eating candy, your natural tendency is to repeat or recreate the experience as often as possible. There is also the tendency for you to seek ways in which to intensify the experience, which further internalizes its effects.

After a while, the urge you feel to continually engage in this pleasant experience becomes a habit. Continued engagement can quickly escalate into a full-blown addiction. This is how your addictive dragon takes birth - right under your nose and with your eyes wide open.

One of nature's unvarying laws is that exercise and regular use of something will strengthen, whereas lack of exercise and lack of use will tend to atrophy. In other words, the more you pursue, engage in, and become obsessed with a type of experience – such as excessive consumption of sugar products – the more apt you are to continue doing so.

The same principle applies to muscular development. When a muscle is exercised regularly it will grow in size and strength. If the same muscle is not used or exercised often it will weaken and possibly atrophy after continual lack of use. The mind acts along the same principle.

One thing is certain: your addictive sugar dragon is born and reared somewhere around the time you develop a strong mental, emotional or physical attachment to the pleasure you get from the excessive consumption of sugar. A person in the early stages of sugar addiction begins eating progressively greater quantities of sugar-rich products, not realizing or caring that the natural digestive mechanism for metabolizing blood sugar primarily for heat and energy is not working properly.

Soon B vitamins - that are crucial for the digestion of sugar - and certain essential minerals such as potassium, calcium, iron, chlorine and sulphur, become deficient. Your body begins to leech B vitamins and these mineral salts - particularly organic calcium - from your body. In time this will result in numerous neurological and metabolic disturbances throughout your body.

Your burgeoning sugar bingeing compromises the structural integrity and function of the pancreas and adrenals. Body cells are unable to complete metabolic functions efficiently due to low nerve force and a chronic condition of ever-increasing cellular waste material that cannot be adequately removed from your cells.

This enervated, toxic condition allows for the eventual breakdown of certain organic and systemic functions. It's at this point that various dangerous, even life-threatening, symptom complexes such as hypoglycemia, diabetes mellitus, and circulatory disorders, can lay claim to your body.

Research has shown that refined sugar and starch addiction is often prevalent where there is a continual lack of energy, willpower, emotional stability, regulated hormone production, over-taxed endocrine glands, and low self-esteem. Education about proper diet, lifestyle modification, and a determined effort to recover are the best preventive measures against continued sugar and starch addiction and habitual bingeing.

The Hidden How and Why of Sugar-Related Mood Swings

One school of current medical thought tends to focus primarily on the role of neurotransmitters - organic chemicals and hormones that carry nervous impulses across nerve synapses such as dopamine and serotonin - in controlling and altering moods.
The leading proponents theorize that when your serotonin receptors are working properly you tend to feel good, upbeat and energetic. You tend to experience restful sleep, and you digest and assimilate food more efficiently due to a more responsive nervous system. When serotonin levels are abnormally low you can feel depressed, enervated, experience insomnia, and your digestive tract may not perform up to par.

Serotonin (5–hydroxytryptophan) is thought to be synthesized in the brain and the digestive tract from the essential amino acid L–tryptophan. Serotonin, in turn, is the "parent" of melatonin, a hormone which helps regulate healthy sleep patterns. Rapid and sudden drops in serotonin levels can cause irritability, anxiety, depression and unclear thought patterns. Although stimulants such as coffee, chocolate, sugar and processed carbohydrates can cause a release of mood-enhancing serotonin, the effect quickly wears off, the serotonin level drops again, and you subsequently crave another hit of sugar, chocolate, etc., to feel good again.

Another serotonin-related factor is stress. High emotional stress can release the hormone cortisol from the adrenal glands. Any dramatic increase in the presence of cortisol in the bloodstream will stimulate a corresponding upward spike in serotonin levels. When cortisol and serotonin levels decrease, you are left with a limp, listless feeling, bordering on enervation and fatigue.

Dr. Bernard Jensen carried out a number of interesting experiments with patients, relating to sugar consumption. His findings revealed that the more sugar patients consumed, the more susceptible they were to bouts of depression, mania, anxiety and paranoia, and the less likely they were to eat healthy, wholesome foods containing essential minerals, vitamins, low-starch carbohydrates, protein and fatty acids.

Jensen further determined that dramatic mood swings and extreme emotional states brought on by overconsumption of sugar products are, more often than not, directly attributed to mineral imbalances in the body. In addition to the well-known vitamin B-depleting effects of excess sugar consumption on the body, Jensen discovered that one or more of the following minerals were often deficient when sugar-related mood swings and erratic emotional states were evident: calcium, chlorine, iron, magnesium, manganese, potassium, and sulfur.

Each area of conscious expression in your life has a corresponding physical brain center that must be fed the proper balance of biochemical elements daily to ensure optimal function. When you regularly consume healthy foods, beverages and whole-food supplements that deliver a wide assortment of essential nutrients, and when you live by natural laws, you will have a direct and telling impact on your physical, mental and emotional life.

Once you begin to live your life by the timeless, commonsense principles of nature's immutable laws of right living, right mindfulness and whole-being health and wellness, this is the point at which you will take the first positive steps toward freeing yourself from the powerful clutches of the addictive sugar dragon and break out of the sugar prison.

And do not think for a moment that nature will nature will not appreciate your efforts. The exact moment you begin to make a strong and sustained effort to free yourself from the dragon's influence and escape from the sugar prison - and from *all* self-imposed prisons - nature will help and support you. She will help you begin laying a strong foundation upon which you can build whole-being health and wellness to last a lifetime.

Should Refined Sugar Be Classified as a Drug?

According to a number of knowledgeable sources, refined sugar should be classified as a drug. Virtually all of the leading alternative health practitioners and nutritional researchers today share this position.

Studies show that refined sugar can be every bit as habit-forming as cocaine, cigarette smoking or alcohol. The fact that little attention is directed to its widespread abuse in the U.S. clearly demonstrates how this ticking time bomb has the potential to cause great devastation in the lives of unwary Americans. Sugar abuse and addiction may soon replace cigarette smoking, drugs and alcohol as America's most serious addictive habit.

Not-so-sweet Criminals

In a landmark study conducted by criminologist Stephen J. Schoenthaler, inmates at a Virginia jail facility were separated into two groups. Group A was fed healthy foods and had sugar-laden foods and desserts for six months. Group B was fed healthy food but no heavy processed sugar products for the same period of time.

During the trial, both groups were equally monitored for stress levels, depression, emotional outbursts and other speech-related and behavioral indicators. After the six-month trial was complete the results of the study indicated that Group B had far fewer behavioral or verbal confrontations with other inmates than Group A. This study was conducted at a number of jail facilities where the results reported matched the original findings.
The news of Schoenthaler's success spread quickly throughout the penal system in Virginia and elsewhere. In ten years Schoenthaler included over 8000 criminal delinquents in his sugar trials.

The steady decrease in sugar consumption, with a concurrent increase in nutritious meals and food supplements, led to a sharp decrease in incidents of physical and verbal violence, escape, depression and suicide attempts. Prisoners were said to have adopted more congenial mindsets and tended to get along with others to a marked degree.

Clearly the evidence suggests that refined sugar had as dramatic an effect on the moods, mindsets and behavior of inmates involved in the trials as many recreational and prescription drugs may have had under similar experimental circumstances.

Sugar Bingeing Rats

In a May 26, 2005, ABC News story *"Studying The Sweet Tooth,"* Schoenthaler's research was corroborated by the findings of Bart Hoebel, a Princeton University professor of psychology. During a series of experiments with rats, he found that refined sugar seemed to have unique addictive properties. After feeding a group of rats a sugar-rich diet, they showed signs of chemical dependency on sugar.

Hoebel and others have been studying the addictive properties of sugar on rats for some years. What he and other researchers have found is that it is not the sugar that is addictive, it is the high it causes – the feeling of temporary euphoria and well-being. Like many drugs, sugar stimulates the release of dopamine, a neurotransmitter that tends to make humans and rats feel good. Hoebel's team determined that, just as with humans, after a sugary meal the rats experienced a release of dopamine, and that their opioid - morphine/opium - receptors were activated.

Within a few days, the rats were "hooked" on the sugar. Reportedly, they each wanted to ingest greater quantities of sugar with each passing day. Their brains created more dopamine receptors. After a month of this regimen, when the sugar was removed, or when the dopamine was chemically blocked using a drug, anxiety increased in the rats, to the point that their teeth chattered audibly - a sign of withdrawal.

When the rats were once again fed, after being deprived of sugar for a few days, they ingested even more, showing a tendency to crave it. Hoebel said that, as you find with addicts, the crucial next step is where the rats learned to binge on sugar.

He further remarked that by day 20, whenever the rats received sugar they consumed a lot, all at once, which was his definition of bingeing.

Although Hoebel's study was conducted with rats, it points to the conclusion that the drug-like addictive effects of sugar have as powerful an effect on lower animals as they do on humans.

CHAPTER 2

More Sugar Woes and Lows

The Dangerous Affinity of Sugar to Calcium

Calcium is leached from your body in direct proportion to how much sugar you consume beyond your body's sensible requirements. Dr. A.D. Birchard, in *Philosophy of Health Magazine*, told of an experiment he conducted. He found that one thousand parts of water could dissolve one part of calcium. When sugar was added to the same amount of water he was able to dissolve 35 times more calcium. You can imagine the incredible leeching ability unutilized sugar has on calcium in your blood stream, lymph, bones and other body parts. This is exactly why infants should not be fed sugars and starches prior to when their bodies are able to begin oxidizing carbohydrates, which usually does not begin to happen until the first set of teeth come in. Otherwise sugar will wreak havoc in the youngster's body.

When a child's teeth do come in, is no time to let down your guard. Actually, this is when sugar addiction and abuse usually starts. Children who consume excessive quantities of sugars and starches can experience "growing pains," toothache, poor bone structure and lack of confidence. Parents notice sores do not heal properly or completely, their children exhibit sporadic bursts of energy and then an inexplicable lack of same shortly thereafter. These are all indications of blood sugar instability and calcium shortage in the body. Children learn that candy, soda pop, cakes and cookies all seem to make them feel better and give them a short, but appreciated, energy boost.

Unfortunately, the mind being the creature of habit that it is, will pursue this dangerous course of energy and feeling enhancement until nature holds up a red flag. This will often come in the form of an unexpected and often serious illness. And this will depend on the degree to which your body has been compromised by carbonosis - a pathological condition where the body becomes overburdened with carbohydrates due to excessive consumption of refined sugars and starches. The result is the body's inability to efficiently oxidize and metabolize sugars.

Soft Drinks and Sugar Substitutes

Whenever there is a discussion on the positive and negative effects of sugar, someone will usually ask: "Are most commercial soft drinks and sugar substitutes bad for you?" I tell them to remove the question mark and slightly shift the position of the words. The result: *Most commercial soft drinks and sugar substitutes are bad for you.*

Your body can only effectively process, digest, assimilate and metabolize organic food-related matter from a plant or animal source. It cannot effectively do any of that with *any* substance it regards as inorganic or hostile to the organism as a whole. The damaging effects of processed sugar products and chemical-based sugar substitutes are often undetectable for years after heavy consumption. Many soft drink products have chemical additives such as emulsifiers, anti-foaming agents, artificial flavors and artificial colors that can compound and exacerbate the negative effects of excessive sugar and starch consumption. Among the more serious side effects can be diabetes, circulatory disorders, kidney ailments, liver damage, glandular system impairment, metabolic imbalance, muscular weakness, chronic constipation, insomnia and neurological disturbances.

Learn to eat wisely and in moderation and you should have no need to supplement your diet with questionable sugar substitutes or other sweeteners. One widely used sugar substitute is made from a combination of two amino acids and ethanol – wood alcohol. The FDA labels ethanol as a poison to the human body.

In an article entitled *"Sugar in the Morning, Sugar in the Evening, Sugar at Suppertime,"* staff writer for *FDA Consumer*, John Henkel, explored issues and suppositions regarding sugar substitutes. Some of the findings include:

- The average American eats the equivalent of 20 teaspoons of sugar a day, according to figures from the most recent federal "Continuing Survey of Food Intakes by Individuals."

- Approximately 60% of this daily sugar intake is from corn sweeteners (such as high fructose corn syrup) used in soft drinks and other sweetened drinks.

- The remaining 40% is from sucrose (table sugar), and a small amount comes from other sweeteners, such as honey and molasses.

- Adam Drewnowski, Ph.D., director of nutritional science at the University of Washington, notes: "Because sugar substitutes, also called artificial sweeteners, are many times sweeter than sugar, it takes much less of them to create the same sweetness."

- According to a 1998 survey by the Calorie Control Council, 144 million American adults regularly consumed low-calorie, sugar-free products such as artificially sweetened sodas and desserts.

- The granddaddy of all sugar substitutes is saccharin. It is 300 times sweeter than sugar. An early attempt to ban saccharin came in 1911 when a board of federal scientists called the artificial sweetener "an adulterant" that should not be used in foods. This same board later decided to limit saccharin to products "intended for invalids" - a restriction that was lifted after World War I began.

- David Hattan, Ph.D., acting director of FDA's division of health effects evaluation, says that aspartame ingestion results in the production of methanol, formaldehyde and formate - substances that could be considered toxic at high doses.

- Other circulating reports claim that two amino acids in aspartame - phenylalanine and aspartic acid - can cause neurotoxic effects such as brain damage. Women with certain genetic traits (e.g., phenylketonurics) may metabolize the amino acid phenylalanine poorly and thus accumulate far higher than normal blood levels of phenylalanine. During pregnancy, high maternal levels of blood phenylalanine can be transferred to the fetus and produce serious adverse effects on brain development.

- Acesulfame potassium: First approved in 1988 as a tabletop sweetener, acesulfame potassium, also called Sunett, is now approved for products such as baked goods, frozen desserts, candies, and, most recently, beverages. About 200 times sweeter than sugar and calorie free, acesulfame potassium often is combined with other sweeteners.

- Sucralose: Also known by its trade name, Splenda, sucralose is 600 times sweeter than sugar. It is bulked up with maltodextrin, a starchy powder, so it will measure more like sugar. It has good shelf life and doesn't degrade when exposed to heat. Numerous studies have shown that sucralose does not affect blood glucose levels, making it an option for diabetics.

- Sugar alcohols: Though not technically considered artificial sweeteners, sugar alcohols are slightly lower in calories than sugar and do not promote tooth decay or cause a sudden increase in blood glucose. They include sorbitol, xylitol, lactitol, mannitol, and maltitol and are used mainly to sweeten sugar-free candies, cookies, and chewing gums.

- Though sugar substitutes have a long history of controversy, the Calorie Control Council says Americans are continually searching for good-tasting, low-calorie products as part of a healthy lifestyle. Market surveys show that calorie-conscious consumers want more low-calorie foods and beverages.

The FDA freely admits there can be serious health risks associated with the regular consumption of sugar substitutes. However, as a rule, they tend to paraphrase their initial pronouncements by adding qualifying statements to the effect that, although a sugar substitute can be hazardous to health in laboratory studies, there is no real-world substantial proof of a given sugar substitute posing a health risk to humans. I caution you to not base your decision to use any sugar substitutes on the FDA's questionable logic or research findings. When it comes to adding an unnatural food item to your daily diet, do your homework. A wrong decision here could cost you dearly.

I do not believe in the long-term use of the great majority of sugar substitutes on the market for a number of reasons not covered in the FDA's research findings. My research has proven that natural, unprocessed sugars, as obtained directly from fruits, vegetables, raw honey and certain grains, are the safest option to pursue where optimal nutrition is concerned.

The Case of the Dissolving Tooth

If you have an addiction or unhealthy attraction to nutritionally poor foods and beverages, you may be seriously compromising your body's cellular integrity. A case in point: nationally renowned nutritional researcher Dr. Clive McCay, longtime professor of nutrition at Cornell University, conducted an experiment, which clearly demonstrated the destructive capabilities of a common soft drink on the skeletal system.

McCay placed a human tooth in a glass filled with a cola soft drink. After only two days the tooth began to decay. Imagine what can happen to the integrity of your entire skeletal structure when you flood your body daily with these kinds of drinks for years on end.

The high phosphoric acid content in many soft drinks can restrict the assimilation of iron by the cells. Another danger not widely discussed in nutritional circles is that overconsumption of commercial soft drinks can expose the liver to cirrhosis.

The types of sugars and chemicals used in most soft drinks and many of the popular sugar substitutes being consumed today are treated as antigens when they enter the digestive system and subsequently the blood stream. Your cells cannot, for the most part, use the sugars made available and they tend to overburden the liver, pancreas, adrenals, kidneys and thyroid.

Any chemicals present in the soft drinks or sugar substitutes will not be metabolized at the cellular level, which means they will be treated as foreign matter. This enters into the overall composition of cellular waste and will often sit tucked away in your cells, joints, intercellular spaces, arterial walls, lymphatics, fatty tissue and other locations for decades, where they can cause untold mischief.

CHAPTER 3

Getting Your Motor Running

A Simple and Effective Dietary Program to Help You Reverse Your Sugar Addiction

Now that you understand how excessive sugar consumption undermines your health, are you ready to do something about it? Will you commit at least a few minutes of your time, every day, for the next couple of months, toward the goal of freeing yourself from your addiction to sugar? If you are, we have a surefire and intelligent game plan that can help you reach your goal.

First step is to counteract the effects of carbonosis. Carbonosis creates a lack of available oxygen and a deficiency of essential biochemical elements and other nutrients. Particularly sodium phosphate, copper, iron and the B complex vitamins required to handle excess carbon dioxide and carbonic acid waste resulting from sugar fermentation.

This condition creates systemic acids and fatty tissue throughout your body. Hardened mucous begins to form in the lungs, blood, lymph and elsewhere in the body. This, in turn, slows nerve force. At that point metabolic function is inefficient, cells become starved for nutrients and energy and the amount of cellular waste increases to the extent that cellular activity is dangerously impaired.

This is when your sugar addiction starts to get serious: it has led to the disease state (toxicosis or toxemia) that ushers in a host of symptom complexes such as diabetes mellitus, hypoglycemia, osteoporosis, cancer, arthritis and other serious conditions. Your sugar dragon has made sure your body will be nutritionally compromised, dysfunctional and, ultimately, most vulnerable to the dragon's continuing influence.

What will you do? Who will you turn to? Not to worry. This is a game you can win if you really *want* to win.

Starting Sensibly

Any dietary and lifestyle modification program to help reverse the damage done to you by excessive sugar consumption must include two sensible components:

1. Realization and acceptance of the fact that you do have a sugar addiction or, at least, a tendency to overindulge in carbohydrate consumption to the detriment of your health.
2. Acknowledgement that you need to reverse your thought and behavior patterns from self-destructive to constructive activities and finding a program of health restoration you can embrace with faith and confidence.

In Part Three you will be introduced to a daily, nutritionally sound regimen that can help cleanse your body and simultaneously allow it to rest while you feed it essential nutrients needed to begin the process of cellular rejuvenation. It will allow your newly awakening body every opportunity to throw off toxic waste material that may have been pent up in your body for years.

While you are cleansing, rejuvenating and rebuilding your body is an excellent time to do the same with your mind. In Part Two you will learn how your mind can keep pace with the reconstruction and rejuvenation of your physical body. It is essential for you to employ both the mindfulness and nutritional aspects of this protocol simultaneously, starting from the first day.

PART TWO

Mindfulness: The Basic States System

CHAPTER 4

Mindfulness: Break Through Your Sugar Addiction and More!

Mindfulness is about being extraordinarily attentive to what arises within your own mind and body and all that presents itself in your life in this very moment. It also involves an accepting, non-judgmental way of being with your thoughts, emotions and physical body sensations.

Mindfulness can help you break out of the sugar prison. It can also help you break out of other mind-body prisons. It turns out that the sugar prison contains within it, all kinds of emotional and psychological prisons. The great power of mindfulness is its applicability to any form of suffering. Any time you are trapped, overwhelmed or controlled by your thoughts, emotions and physical sensations, mindfulness can be applied.

The situations amenable to mindfulness practice need not be tragic, dramatic or even overwhelming. Minor irritations, frustration, confusion, aches, pains, jealousy and other destructive behaviors aside from sugar addiction are all amenable to mindfulness practice. It is a generic solution to the issue of human suffering.

It usually seems as though people, places, things and situations are your problem in life. This is actually not the case. The real problem is your relationship to the thoughts, feelings and body discomforts that are triggered by the people, places and situations. Once you begin a thorough exploration of your mind and body using mindfulness methods, you will realize that thoughts, feelings and body discomforts, in and of themselves, can be greatly reduced as problematic experiences. Then you can deal with challenging life situations with greater ease.

Mindfulness is a new and radical concept that you will experience and clarify as you read on. You will see that the major point of mindfulness practice is to *transform your relationship* to your mind/body states to one that is gentle and accepting. Then suffering will decrease even if you can't alter the situations. You then become a person who is not controlled by pleasure and pain. This point carries a lot of weight in helping you out of the sugar prison as well as other mind/body prisons since all of your prisons involve pleasure and pain and the difficulty you have managing these states. The technique you will learn in this section of the book is known as the "Basic States" method of mindfulness. It will show you what your destructive urges are really about and ways to break free of them. In order to break free of destructive urges you must see how these urges fit into the picture of what we call "suffering."

CHAPTER 5

What is Suffering?

Hatred

You are often times quite aggressive towards yourself. You hate your unpleasant feelings, you hate your troubled thinking and you hate the way your body feels when it's uncomfortable. With mindfulness you will come to realize and directly experience the fact that hatred (aversion) towards the discomfort experienced in the mind and body is the real problem rather than the discomfort itself. The hatred towards your mind/body is one type of relationship that keeps you imprisoned. It is the hatred towards your uncomfortable sugar desires that causes you to suffer. You then relieve the suffering by acting out the negative destructive behavior of eating sugar. A very important point to realize is that no matter how hard you try, *you will never be able to avoid discomfort*. Mindfulness offers you the opportunity to learn how to uncover a sense of freedom in the midst of unpleasant mind and body states so they don't have to control your behavior.

Clinging

Clinging (craving) is another aspect of the suffering problem. The desire to hold on to pleasure gets in the way of your peacefulness and is directly related to your sugar addiction. You think of the candy bar and pleasure fills your body. Wanting pleasure is different from craving it. Craving is associated with a strong urge or "I have to" experience. So you feel as though you have to go out and get a donut and it tastes so good and then you want more and you go out and get more, and so on and so forth. A very important point to keep in mind is that *pleasure never lasts. It always passes and then you suffer.*

If craving has a physiological basis, the nutritional program outlined in this book can help reduce craving. However, almost certainly, you will need to work with the emotions and thoughts that drive the compulsion. Mindfulness offers you powerful tools to decrease and eliminate craving, whether your issue is emotional, physical or a combination of both.

Sugar addiction and other forms of addiction involve an interplay between aversion to discomfort and craving for pleasure. These two human tendencies cause suffering. Then you seek out the sugar drug for the very temporary relief of your suffering. You reach for the drug that numbs you. The relief is *only for a moment then the moment's gone!*

Mindfulness teaches you to how to decrease or eliminate both craving and aversion. You learn to replace these negative human tendencies with what we call "equanimity." This is a loving, gentle, accepting way of relating to your mind and body experiences. You neither hold on to pleasure nor push away pain. This type of relationship will literally unravel your suffering and lead to permanent life transformation. The process of unraveling involves learning to open up to your internal experience. This allows pain and pleasure to just do its own dance while changing and passing naturally. When you're not caught up in your mind/body process, you are less likely to engage in negative, self-destructive behaviors to relieve your anguish.

Unconsciousness

The third cause of suffering is unconsciousness. Here's an analogy: Let's say that you are ill and have various symptoms but you don't know what's wrong with you. You go to a doctor and the doctor says: "I'm aware of your symptoms but in order to help you cure the illness, I need to investigate your condition further. I'd like you to have x-rays and blood tests and then come back for another appointment." So you have the x-rays and blood tests and you go back to the doctor. The doctor says, "OK. I put your blood under a microscope and I've looked at your x-rays carefully. Now I can give you the appropriate medicine to cure your illness." Before the doctor thoroughly investigated your condition, no help could be offered.

It's a similar situation with mindfulness and your issues of anguish. Mindful awareness involves putting your mind/body process under the microscope of extraordinary focus, and bringing a non-judgmental, radical acceptance to the experience. This type of awareness, in and of itself is the medicine that cures, or at least lessens the suffering, i.e. the bother and imposition that your mind/body has on your sense of well-being. This type of awareness relieves you of the hatred and clinging that accompanies your reactions.

You'll understand this better when you begin to experience it with the exercises set out for you in this book. It's important to remember that while working with your sugar addiction or any form of suffering, you must become aware of what's going on below the surface of ordinary consciousness or nothing significant can be done about your anguish. Think back to the doctor analogy. The doctor couldn't do anything for the patient until the condition was investigated thoroughly.

Here's how unconsciousness leads to suffering when it involves sugar addiction. Sugar addiction is characterized by strong desire. You feel compelled to consume it. Consider for a moment, the times when you feel as though you have to eat sugar. The sense of "I have to" or of being driven is a form of suffering that manifests as bother or disturbance.

Again, it's like being in prison because you've lost the power to control your own behavior. In that moment of performing the behavior, you aren't conscious of *why* you have the compulsive urge to do it. You may be thinking, "I'll go nuts if I don't have a cookie now." Maybe there is also a sensation of anxiety somewhere in your stomach. Maybe in that moment your mouth is watering. Maybe you are going through sugar withdrawals. Maybe there are mental pictures in your mind of your favorite cookies. However, in that moment of "I have to" you are unconscious of all those specifics I just mentioned and you certainly are not relating to them in a mindful way. Your experience is only; "I have to do it". Then you are on automatic pilot - unconsciousness. Automatic pilot masks the internal processes occurring within the experience of "I have to" or compulsion.

Mindfulness decreases or eliminates unconsciousness in the following way. You shine the light of your own awareness on the mind/body processes with the focusing methods you will learn and you cease fighting with these mind/body processes. The two qualities of mindful awareness, that is, extraordinary attentiveness and acceptance, eliminate your internal war allowing the urge to decrease or completely dissolve. Then you won't need to seek something outside yourself to alleviate the discomfort.

Mindful awareness helps you to open up and allow thoughts and feelings to just pass through rather than get stuck. Compulsive urges, even those feeling like solid icebergs, can literally dissolve in minutes *if* you have the willingness and courage to stay mindful of them for however long it takes. No one can predict how much time will be needed for them to pass, but as you practice the mindfulness methods, the amount of time needed gets shorter and your tolerance for experiencing the negative urges grows stronger.

CHAPTER 6

Lightening the Weight

Divide and Conquer

One of the unique and powerful principles of the Basic States method is known as "Divide and Conquer." Let's imagine that your issue of suffering is craving for sugar and it weighs 100 lbs. That's a heavy weight to pick up. If you were to break down that 100-lb. weight into 25-lb pieces, it would be much, much easier to pick up 25 lbs. four times rather than the entire 100-lb weight all at once. The Basic States method helps you break down the weight of your experiences of suffering, such as destructive urges, into smaller and more manageable mind/body components.

Let's say your desire for sugar involves mental pictures (a chocolate donut), verbal internal dialog (I have to have that), and emotional body sensations (fear in your gut). The experience weighs 100 lbs. Being mindful of one component at a time, decreases or eliminates the suffering within that component. Then that component of experience has less power over you. If the weight of one component is lightened, then the entire weight is lightened. Since the urge is made up of those specific components the weight of the urge itself is made lighter. Now there is a decrease or elimination of the sense of being compelled to act out the destructive behavior.

Mindfulness can help you to experience an urge with less or no bother, overwhelm or sense of powerlessness. The same is true for anxiety, grief, sadness, pain, etc.

CHAPTER 7

The Basics of Mindfulness Practice

Concentration, Clarity and Equanimity

Mindful awareness has three basic components. One is concentration. Research supports the fact that mindfulness can lead to profound states of concentration (*Time*, 2003). Concentration will not only help you with the skill needed to work with your sugar addiction but also with your experiences of daily life. Consider an activity or experience in your life that is particularly meaningful for you. It could be any experience such as work, study, play, hobbies, etc. You have probably noticed that sometimes during that activity, you become very focused and "present" while other times you are less focused and present. You have probably also noticed that when you are more focused, the activity is more fulfilling or effective and when you are less focused the activity is not as fulfilling or effective. Mindfulness practice allows you to be optimally focused during all your activities.

Few people realize that states of high concentration can be developed with systematic practice. It is a skill that will bring improvements over the entire spectrum of your life while also helping you with your sugar urges. Concentration comes with repeated practice of the techniques along with mindfulness in action. If practicing the methods becomes part of your daily regimen, you can build strength in a similar manner to developing muscle strength. The more consistent your workouts at the gym, the stronger your muscles become.

You must develop concentration in order to have clarity of your internal experience. Concentration power brings about the mental clarity that is necessary to engage in the divide-and-conquer process. Mental clarity is extremely necessary to eliminate the unconsciousness that I spoke about earlier. The doctor needed to put your blood under a microscope to see what was *really* going on. Then the illness could be cured. All the methods that you will learn in this section of the book will involve the development of concentration and clarity.

The other basic component of mindful awareness is known as equanimity. Equanimity is a powerful and fundamental skill for self-examination. It's a subtle, deep concept that can easily be misunderstood or confused with lack of expressiveness, apathy or suppression. The simplest definition would be "inner balance." Equanimity does not come about by trying to squelch your thoughts, feelings or other discomforts, but rather by opening up to them and allowing them to arise, spread and pass naturally.

Other ways of describing equanimity are acceptance rather than rejection — non-judgmental awareness, opening rather than freezing, loving rather than hateful, softening rather than tightening, or making peace with oneself. Practicing the methods is like training, and equanimity becomes natural over time. You can also create it by relaxing tight jaws, allowing your tense body to go limp, and just observing your sensory experiences.

CHAPTER 8

The Significance of Change

Mindfulness and Nature

Now let's explore mindfulness and nature and the importance of change. If you look around outdoors, notice the "just happening" quality of nature. The rain pours, the rivers flow, the flowers bloom and wither, people are born and die and the sun rises and sets. Nothing and no one can stop nature, even though we would often like to. You would never even consider trying to stop the rain or snow from falling or the wind from blowing.

I have a question for you. Are you part of nature? The answer, of course, is yes. You were naturally brought into the world and you will naturally be taken from it. Here's another question. Are your thoughts, feelings and physical sensations part of nature? Again the answer is "yes." As human beings it is natural to have thoughts, emotions and physical sensations. It is part of being alive and human. The problem is that human beings have strong tendencies towards grasping what feels good, and rejecting what feels bad.

If nature is giving you pleasure then it is natural, and if nature is giving you pain, that is also natural. Now you might think, if I break my leg, it's natural to want to get rid of the pain. This is true. However, nature has given you pain for a reason. There is nothing wrong with trying to relieve it. But what if you can't relieve it?

Mindfulness offers you a skill that can allow you to have a sense of well-being even if you can't be rid of the pain or any other type of discomfort. This sense of well-being comes about by opening up and turning towards what's arising within you rather than tensing up and turning away from it. Without the resistance, the problem ceases to get in your way. By training away the resistance to pain, you are not *dependent* on being rid of it for your sense of well-being. This is a new and refreshing way of living your life. Mindfulness offers you a new and amazing way to live!

Nature is change and change is the true nature of all experience and all that exists. This becomes evident as a result of mindfulness practice. Insight into impermanence allows you to experience your mind and body less as a particle and more as a wave. This in turn leads to the experience of fluidity in the mind and body. This is its natural state, even though it may not seem that way at the time.

Mindfulness helps you to become capable of having thoughts, feelings and physical sensations without being overwhelmed or controlled by them since you are just allowing them to arise and pass away as nature has intended. Thus there is an intimate link between change and a deep sense of calm and peacefulness in day-to-day life. With profound concentration and allowing nature to take over within yourself, you literally ride on the wave of the present moment. Change becomes revitalizing since each moment is experienced as fresh with a full range of new possibilities.

"*A flower falls even though we love it and a weed grows even though we don't love it*" - Dogen

CHAPTER 9

Becoming Aware of the Ordinary

The Basic Mind/Body States

The Basic States method is a unique and powerful form of mindfulness training. It involves becoming aware of ordinary, everyday aspects of your daily human experience. Let's look at four of them now. One or more of these four aspects of experience is involved with every part of living. The four states are physical body sensations, emotional body sensations, mental images and your internal, verbal dialog. If you consider your sugar addiction, it could involve withdrawals: these might be physical sensations or possibly emotional sensations like anxiety, and possibly internal dialog such as "I have to eat that now." As you saw in the divide and conquer section, if you bring mindful awareness to one of these components of your experience, lightening the weight of that piece affects the weight of the entire experience.

Labeling (naming)

One of the most significant and powerful aspects of The Basic States method is called "labeling" which is naming your specific mind/body experiences. You will use a different label or name for each state of consciousness that you work with. Labeling is not mandatory for practicing the Basic States method but it is extremely helpful and highly recommended in your formal sitting practice. It is very useful for creating the non-judgmental relationship towards what arises within yourself and getting a more objective view of it. Labeling helps you to "just observe" your experience.

Making labels also helps with staying focused and developing the skill of concentration, which is of utmost importance in this method. This does not mean you will be labeling your experiences as you walk through life but at times you may want to for extra support with difficult or overwhelming internal experiences.

Feel: This is the name you will use to describe body sensations that seem emotional in nature. When you feel bad, most of the time you can notice an unpleasant sensation in your body, and when you feel good, you can notice a pleasant body sensation. These types of sensations are very important to be mindful of since suffering can come from both pleasurable and painful emotional body sensations. This fact is significant because pleasure and pain are involved in your sugar addiction.

Notice that the label "feel" is very non-judgmental and quite neutral. It's not associated with good, bad, right, wrong, pleasure or pain. Using a neutral name for emotional sensation, doesn't make you feel neutral. It engages the left frontal cortex of the brain, so that you can experience your feelings without overwhelm. Then you won't be trapped or controlled by your experience. It's important to remember that you potentially can be equally as controlled by pleasurable emotions as you can by painful emotions.

Image: This is the name for your internal mental pictures of people, places, things or situations. Images can get in the way of your sense of well-being. They don't have to if you just name them with this label "image." Then it's experienced as a mental picture that is not charged up with your own preconceptions, ideas and judgments. You experience it *just as it is* in its basic, naked form.

Talk: This is the label for your internal, verbal dialog or the words in your head. Again, it's a very non-judgmental and matter-of-fact name. This name will help you to just observe the self-talk without holding on to it or pushing it away. The naming helps you to just *let it be* and let nature take its course by allowing it to come and go without the friction and internal disturbance created by craving or aversion.

Touch: This is the label or name for physical, non-emotional body sensation, such as pain, sensing the clothes on your body, tension in your neck, heat, cold, warmth, or your feet touching the floor. Physiological sugar withdrawals and a watering mouth would be examples of physical touches. Both could be very significant when it comes to your sugar addiction. As you may realize, it would be important to acquire an ability to experience these physical sensations in a way that you are not imprisoned by them. Mindfulness teaches you how.

Sight: This is the label or name given to the open-eyed external visual field. Objects in your visual field will be part of a powerful external technique that you will learn. Any objects in your external visual experience will be labeled "sight."

Sound: This is the label given to external sounds. Sound will be part of the external method that you will learn.

Mindfulness is not about rejection of any human experience. It is about meeting and accepting yourself just as you are in that moment. Self-acceptance does not imply that you shouldn't attempt to make changes. It means a complete embracing of your mind and body in that moment. This point is *extremely* important. Again I will emphasize the fact that the labeling used in this mindfulness method will help you have a relationship with your mind/body states that is not characterized by craving, aversion or unconsciousness, which are the three causes of suffering.

Labeling aids you in the process of just noticing your experience. Labeling brings about a welcoming, friendly, gentle and kind relationship with what arises within you. This type of relationship leads to internal peace rather than war. It leads to freedom from the bondage of the mind/body prison.

In the case of your sugar addiction, the sense of well-being brought about through mindfulness, reduces the probability that you will engage in destructive behavior. At the same time, there is nothing wrong with changing circumstances to bring about comfort and happiness. This is a perfectly valid human goal. The difference between the goal of mindfulness and the usual goal of fixing what's broken and being rid of what you hate, is that mindfulness is about *unconditional* freedom. This means that you are not dependent on changing the conditions of your internal or external world for a sense of fulfillment and well-being.

Research

There is a wealth of credible research supporting the power of mindfulness for stress, pain, emotional distress and addictions that include eating issues. One interesting study supports a labeling method for bringing about positive brain changes. A team of researchers at UCLA triggered negative emotions in the subjects. When they compared the brain scans of subjects who had a mindful disposition using a labeling method, to the subjects who were less mindful, they found a stark difference. The mindful subjects experienced greater activation in the ventrolateral-prefrontal cortex (executive, rational center of the brain) and a greater calming effect in the amygdala (emotional center of brain), after labeling their emotions (*Psychosomatic Medicine*, 2007).

In another study, subjects who had done mindfulness showed positive and long-lasting changes in both the brain and immune function (*Psychosomatic Medicine*, 2003). The activation of the left frontal region of the brain, associated with lower anxiety and a more positive emotional state was demonstrated.

Dr. Jean Kristellar, a professor at Indiana State University, has done studies on compulsive eating behavior with attendees of her mindfulness-based program. She found that bingeing behavior was reduced from four to one-and-one-half per week. She replicated the study several times and got similar results. (In Baer, R. (2006) *Mindfulness-based approaches to eating disorders*).

Let's look specifically at basic human experiences and the labels that you will use to describe them when you practice the methods in this book.

CHAPTER 10

The Power of Restful States

Restful States

The Basic States method helps you to access restful states within yourself. How can mindfulness of restful states be helpful? They are important for release of suffering and also for the pleasure of restfulness itself. They can create a positive feedback loop that strengthens your power to concentrate. The more you concentrate on restfulness, the better you feel, motivating you to give even greater concentration to the restful states. These pleasant states also create a kind of container within which the ordinary states such as unpleasant emotions can come and go without causing suffering. In other words, the restful states tend to induce equanimity, i.e. the accepting, non-judgmental, non-violent manner of relating to yourself. This way of relating to your mind and body is one of the central goals of mindfulness practice. As you practice the methods, you'll quickly see how acceptance of your inner experience reduces or eliminates anguish.

Most people fail to notice and enjoy the restful states that are present within the mind and body. The Basic States method gives you the vocabulary and concepts needed to recognize and enjoy them.

Blank: This is the name or label given to one of the restful states. You will be able to observe it when you close your eyes during the restful states exercise. It consists of the brightness and darkness that you experience either in front of or behind your closed eyes.

Relaxed: This is the label given to a sense of being settled or relaxed. This state can be experienced after a good massage. You can always access relaxation even without the massage. Every time you breathe out, notice there is some sense of relaxation. If you tense parts of your body and then release them, you will notice relaxation.

Peace: In the context of the Basic States technique, this name does *not* mean feeling good. It means "emotional neutrality" or "I don't have any emotional body sensations right now."

Quiet: This label signifies the absence of the internal, verbal dialog.

CHAPTER 11

Guided Mindfulness Exercises

Focus In

Techniques number 1 through 3 involve working with the components of your subjective reactions, that is, mental pictures, internal verbal dialog and emotional body sensations.

Technique #1: Focus on Image Space

When you close your eyes, maintain an upright posture and uncross your arms and legs. This allows for alertness and openness. Bring your attention to your closed-eye mental screen, which you will most likely experience in front of or behind your eyes. This is called "image space." If you notice the arising of a mental picture of a person, place, thing or situation, you will say the word "image" to yourself in a gentle internal voice. If you don't notice any images you will say the word "blank" to yourself.

Say your labels slowly to yourself. If your attention is pulled away to the internal dialog, emotional sensations or physical sensations, gently return your attention to image or blank. Don't try to push other experiences away. Image or blank will be present at any given moment. Intently focus your awareness on whichever is present. If it is hard to focus, say your label out loud and listen to your own voice.

Finding it hard to focus is not a negative situation. Think of it as a strength- building exercise such as lifting weights. In the beginning, it might be really challenging, but as you keep lifting the weights, it gets easier and easier. The end result is that you have strong muscles. It's the same with mindfulness practice. There is no right or wrong or good or bad. You are just noticing what is there or what is not there. There is no "should" or "should not." You are just allowing nature to take its course within image space. You either have images or you don't.

Make the label, i.e., say the word to yourself, every few seconds. Even if you have cascades of mental pictures, continue to make your label slowly, spacing your labels apart for a few seconds. Allow pictures to go by in between naming them "image." If you are not sure what is arising, then guess. If you forget the name of the label, just notice your experience.

Here's an example of my personal experience:

"Image, image, blank, image, blank, image"

(Set your timer for 5 minutes and begin)

Technique #2: Focus on Talk Space

When you close your eyes, if you notice any verbal internal dialog arise, say the word "talk" to yourself. If you don't notice any words, make the label "quiet." You might think, "If I say the word quiet to myself, then it is really "talk" because I heard the word talk. This is not the case. It's merely an acknowledgment that you noticed an absence of "talk." You are not labeling the labels. If your attention gets pulled away to images, or emotional or physical body sensations, just let those be in the background and re-focus you attention on to talk space, naming your experience talk or quiet. If at any time you are not sure, then guess.

Here's an example of my personal experience:

"Quiet, quiet, quiet, talk, quiet, talk, talk"

(Set your timer for 5 minutes and begin)

Technique #3: Focus on Feel Space

The definition of "feel" is body sensation that seems emotional in nature to you. Some examples of emotional body sensations are anger, sadness, grief, anxiety, joy, and excitement. If you're not sure whether you are experiencing emotional body sensations, then guess. As you bring awareness to your body, if you notice any sensations that seem emotional in nature, say the word "feel" to yourself. Intently focus on feel if it is present. If your body seems emotionally neutral, then say the word "peace" to yourself and intently focus on peace. Peace doesn't mean feeling good. Feeling good is feel. In this method peace means feeling neutral. If you prefer another term for describing emotional neutrality then use that term.

Here's an example of my personal experience:

"Peace, peace, feel, feel, feel, peace"

(Set your timer for 5 minutes and begin)

These exercises were your first practice session in focusing on your internal reactions and restful states. The ordinary, everyday human reactions (feel, image, talk) are part and parcel of any form of emotional suffering. Focusing on the restful states (peace, blank, quiet) deepens your equanimity (openness and acceptance) thereby helping you handle the ordinary states with more peacefulness and composure, with less or no imposition on your sense of well being. The active states are involved with all experiences, including the suffering issues related to your sugar addiction. This is why it is so important that you learn to relate to them in a way that you are not overwhelmed or controlled by them. With practice, you will naturally live your life this way, since your new habit will take over in a profoundly positive way.

Focus on Rest

Now I would like you to practice with two restful states, "blank" and "relaxation." It's easy, fun and very relaxing.

Technique #4: Focus on Blank

When you close your eyes, bring attention to your closed-eye mental screen. Notice that there is both brightness and darkness on that screen. Now intently and deeply focus *only* on brightness or darkness, whichever you happen to be drawn to in the moment. If image, talk, feel or other experiences pull your attention away, gently bring your focus back to brightness or darkness. Don't try to get rid of other experiences. Just allow them to be in the background and bring your focus back to brightness or darkness. As you do this, you will say the word "blank" to yourself every few seconds intently focusing on blank only.

(Set your timer for 5 minutes and begin)

Technique #5: Focus on Relaxation

As you bring awareness to your body, notice if there's any relaxation in your body. It could be your whole body or maybe a part of your body like an arm or a leg. If you don't notice any relaxation in your body, then notice that on every exhalation there is some sense of relaxation. You can also intentionally create relaxation by dropping your shoulders or loosening a tight jaw. Now intently focus on relaxation and say the word "relaxed" to yourself. From one moment to the next your awareness may shift to different areas of relaxation in your body. If you become aware of thoughts, emotions or other experiences, let those be in the background, and let your focus be on relaxation only. Give yourself completely to relaxation.

Here's an example of my personal experience:

"Relaxed, relaxed, relaxed, relaxed"

(Set your timer for 5 minutes and begin)

Focus Out

The following method involves focusing out, away from your emotional reactions that arise in the feel, image, or talk spaces. It is an eyes-open exercise. It is an easy and useful way to be mindful in your daily activities. It's also useful when you have cravings for sugar or if you are experiencing unpleasant emotional states.

Technique #6: Focus on Touch, Sight, Sound

As you begin this exercise, straighten your spine and have an upright posture. Let your open eyes have a soft gaze. From one moment to the next you'll be drawn to external sights, external sounds or physical touches in the body. You will say "sight" or "sound" or "touch," to yourself, labeling whichever one you are drawn to in that moment. Intently and deeply focus on the state you are drawn to. If you are drawn to more than one at the same time, pick one to focus on — it doesn't matter which. Rather than skim over your experience, intently focus your attention on sights, sounds or touches. Let your awareness float naturally. You may be drawn to one more than the other or maybe the same one for the entire exercise.

Here's an example of my personal experience:

In this moment I see a flower. I will say the word sight to myself. In this moment I am aware of the sound of a jet in the sky, so I will say the word sound to myself. In this moment I am noticing a dog on a leash, so I will say the word sight to myself. At this moment I am aware of the sweat on my skin, so I will say touch to myself.

For example:

"Sight, sight, sight, sound, touch, sight, sound, sound"

(Set your timer for 5 minutes and begin)

In the methods you have learned here, there is the option to label the state that arises in your awareness in any given moment. You may choose not to use the label. In that case, just observe it. You also have the option to speak your labels out loud or remain silent.

Now that you have practiced the mindfulness methods I've presented, choose your favorite technique, and practice it for 10 minutes.

Your choices are as follows:

1. Feel space (feel or peace)
2. Image space (image or blank)
3. Talk space (talk or quiet)
4. Blank (brightness or darkness)
5. Relaxed (relaxation in the body
6. Touch, sight, sound (physical sensations, external sights, external sounds)

Stay with the technique you have chosen for the entire exercise. If you get pulled away to another space, gently return your awareness to your original technique

CHAPTER 12

Getting the Most Out of Mindfulness - The Basic States Method

Sitting Practice

A formal sitting practice is an important part of learning the skill of mindfulness. It is an opportunity to face yourself without distractions. This is how you root out the deepest poison and pain within yourself, which of course is part of your sugar addiction and all other forms of addiction and suffering. Sitting practice will help you get the most out of mindfulness because it is equivalent to playing scales on a piano with the intent of becoming a concert pianist. If you practice scales every day, by the time you play at a concert, your experience has taken over and is completely natural. It is exactly the same with mindfulness training. You practice the techniques and you naturally become a person who can walk through life with all of its ups and downs, maintaining a sense of ease and peacefulness.

Practice in Action

Practice in action refers to your strategy for maintaining mindfulness in the midst of ordinary daily activities. It is also of utmost importance in getting the most out of mindfulness. It is what you do to keep up a momentum of mindfulness between periods of formal practice. One of the easiest and most natural ways is the "touch, sight, sound" method. In all of your activities, one or more of these three states is in your awareness. It's not necessary to use the labels all of the time, but you may want to choose certain times to do a labeling in action practice. Labeling can be useful when you have a challenging emotion arise in your life. If this happens, you just allow the emotional reaction to be there, and continue to bring awareness back to touch, sight or sound. As a general mindfulness in action practice, you remain attentive to what you see, what you hear and the touches involved with what you do.

Another easy way to practice mindfulness in action if you are having an emotional challenge is to focus on "feel." You maintain a background awareness of your body, just relaxing into feel. You stay with feel even if images or talk arise. Just keep returning awareness to feel until it dissolves or becomes completely manageable. It is extremely important during both sitting and action practice to return awareness to your technique when other experiences draw your attention away. This is how you build strength and build new pathways in the brain.

In the Appendix, you will find the Daily Mindfulness For Life Worksheet. The worksheet will serve as a reminder to bring mindfulness practice into your daily life activities. For best results, write out the answers to the questions at the end of each day. .or read the entire sheet at the end of each day. If you read the sheet at the beginning of the day, it can serve as a reminder of potential pitfalls.

CHAPTER 13

Abstaining from Sugar Bingeing

Practicing Mindfulness with Sugar Cravings

The Touch, Sight, Sound method, also known as "Focus Out," is very useful for working with sugar cravings as well as any difficult mind/body disturbance. Since application of this method is working in a neutral arena - rather than feel, image, and talk - it tends to allow for a very grounding experience. The Focus Out method grounds you in external reality so that you can maintain mindful awareness even in the midst of the significant challenge.

If you choose this method when the cravings come up, you must stay focused only on touch, sight or sound until the cravings disappear or you no longer feel driven by them. Everything within you will want to grab onto the thoughts of the sugary food and escape from the feelings associated with the sugar craving. You must stay focused on touch, sight or sound at this time. If you get pulled away into feel, image or talk, return your awareness to touch, sight or sound. You must stay with the technique in order to break through the negative urge. By "breaking through" I mean allowing it to change and pass away. It is here that you must take a stand! In the Basic States method you must dive off the cliff into the unknown to break out of the sugar prison. One bite can send you back to prison. There are some eating disorder programs that work on helping people to "just have one." If you feel that you are one of those people, you can find a program that suits you and still make use of mindfulness. However, the emphasis of this book is complete abstinence from refined sugar, since the majority of sugar addicts cannot control their consumption.

The dissolution of your craving does *not* mean that you are cured of your sugar addiction. You are in the process of changing significant brain pathways but you cannot eliminate some of them. You will always have the predisposition for sugar bingeing behavior. You are most likely a person who must entirely eliminate refined sugar from your life. When sugar is out of your life, you are then "in life" in a way that you could never have dreamed possible.

Another strategy for handling sugar cravings or difficult emotions would be focusing only on "touch" or only on "feel." or "sight" or "sound". This restriction of awareness to one state keeps it simple. Any method you choose is fine. The most important point is that you stay with the method until your compulsion or emotional discomfort dissolves or loses its power.

In the midst of a compulsive urge you may also focus on rest. If you can sit down at that time, you can focus on blank or relaxed. If you are not able to sit you can focus on relaxation by noticing your exhale, dropping your shoulders, or finding a specific area of the body that feels relaxed. This may not be as easy as using the focus out methods or the focus on feel method, but try it and see how it works for you.

Again, YOUR SUCCESS with emotional issues, which includes compulsive urges, *totally* depends on your willingness to stay with the technique you have chosen until the suffering or urge becomes manageable or is eliminated. If you are unable to stay with the urge until it passes then stay with it for as long as you can. This is still good and any amount of time that you remain with the urge is better than nothing. This way of practicing with your sugar urges or actually any negative urge, will lead to permanent transformation over time.

CHAPTER 14

Eating as a Meditation

Working Through Compulsion and Elevating Satisfaction

By Shinzen Young

If you should happen to be a food addict as well as a sugar addict, you want to be sure to include eating meditation as part of your daily routine. Researchers who studied a mindfulness-based eating disorder program, found that the strongest predictor of improvement in eating control was the amount of time the subjects engaged in eating-related mindfulness (Baer, R., 2006). The following is a description along with instruction for an eating meditation written by Shinzen Young. The focus of the eating meditation is the touch and feel states. Smell and taste would be considered touch.

Each time you take a bite, taste sensations spread over your palate, tongue, cheeks and throat, and smell spreads into your nose. If the tastes are pleasant, it will cause a rippling of pleasant sensation through your body. An analogy may be helpful: When a pebble is tossed into a pond, it causes a splash where it lands, and from that splash ripples spread through the whole pond. The morsel of food is like the pebble; your body is like the pond. The explosion of tastes in your mouth is the splash and the associated reaction of your whole body is the rippling. This global reaction may be subtle, but remember, when it comes to working with feeling, subtle is significant. If you can detect the ripples and let them come and go without clenching, you will greatly deepen your sense of satisfaction.

Eating meditation is an example of spiritual purification through experiencing pleasure with extraordinary attentiveness and radical acceptance (equanimity). Through it your baseline of fulfillment in daily life can be permanently elevated. Since it involves a tangible pleasant object of concentration, it makes a good complement to sitting meditation where unpleasant sensations are sometimes present.

Of course, sometimes unpleasant sensations may arise during eating. For example, if you eat something that you dislike, waves of tension, aversion and cringing may spread through your body. Although it is not necessary to seek such an unpleasant experience, it is helpful to remember that by bringing extraordinary attentiveness and radical acceptance to those sensations, deep psychological blockages such as separation, fear and alienation are being broken up.

Eating slowly and mindfully may also cause one to become impatient and driven to gobble. If this should happen, be happy! It represents a significant opportunity to work through the drivenness and achieve more ease in daily life.

If during the eating process, you feel impatient and driven, try to detect this in terms of tangible "driver sensations" throughout your body. What is true of the ripples of pleasant sensation that bring satisfaction is also true of the tensions and pressures that produce drivenness: they may be subtle and cover much or all of your body.

Observe them with precision and acceptance. In this way, drivenness - not only around eating but in all aspects of your life - will get worked through. Life becomes lighter and easier. Your actions become dynamic and zestful, arising from a fundamental inner peace as opposed to being driven by subliminal suffering.

When approaching eating as a form of meditation, it is useful to pay attention to your posture. Try to keep your spine straight while at the same time allowing the whole body to settle in. Rather than meditating while eating, try to get the sense that you are in a deep meditation sit during which you just happen to be eating.

Eating slowly will help you focus and also perhaps bring up driver sensations. In order to deepen your state, you may want to occasionally pause, put down your utensils and close your eyes for a period of time. After you have completed your meal, it is instructive to sit for a while and savor the delicate vibrations of satisfaction that suffuse your body after pleasant experiences. In daily life we seldom have an opportunity to contact this significant phenomenon.

You may find that a rhythm develops as you eat. You are aware of the tactile sensations in your hand and arm as you reach for the food, then the flavor qualities and texture sensations in different parts of your mouth and the smells going up to your nose, then your whole body reacting to the tastes and smells, and finally the gradual subsiding of taste, smell and body reaction. Then the cycle begins again. Drivenness and impatience may arise just before a bite, or as the flavor and pleasure subsides after a bite, or throughout the whole process. Try to love your impatience to death by patiently observing it.

Two sources of distraction during eating meditation are thinking and preoccupation with what is happening around you. Remember, your defined object of mindfulness is taste, smell and body sensations. As soon as you feel the tug outward into the sights and sounds around you, gently return to taste, smell and body sensations. As soon as you feel the tug inward - to planning, judging, fantasizing and memory - lovingly return to taste, smell and body sensation.

If you are willing to put in some effort, you can enter a kind of slow motion - an "eternal present" - while eating. The simplest fare then becomes an extraordinary experience.

CHAPTER 15

Mindfulness to Combat Other Destructive Urges

At the beginning of this book, I mentioned that the good news about mindfulness is its application to all forms of suffering. This includes addictions other than sugar and food. Addictions take many forms. Any "I have to" behavior is an addiction. If you don't have any "I have to" behaviors then chances are that you still have at least one addiction and that is to "thinking." Notice how your thoughts often times have a "sticky gluey" quality about them. Or "having to" have answers can cause significant suffering for individuals.

The following article was written by Shinzen Young regarding the use of mindfulness for negative urges. Negative urges can be involved with work, addictive relationships, smoking, drugs, alcohol, and so on.

Using Mindfulness Practice to Deal with Negative Urges

By Shinzen Young

The basic trick in resisting negative urges is divide and conquer. If we can analyze an urge into its components, it becomes simply the sum of a few basic phenomena, each of which is manageable. Conversely, when we fail to clearly detect these components individually, they crisscross and multiply with each other, producing the illusory impression of an overwhelming compulsion that we cannot resist, despite our best intentions. What then are the natural elements of the urge process which we must learn to detect?

To begin with, part of the urge process usually involves thoughts - memories, plans, judgments, fantasies, wishes or beliefs. Thoughts may take the form of mental conversations with yourself. They may also take the form of mental pictures. Another part of the urge process involves uncomfortable body sensations. Some of these body sensations are more emotional in origin. You may experience the sensations of sadness, irritation, fear, hurt, impatience, agitation, etc. It is important to remember that all emotions consist of a mixture of thoughts and body sensations. The actual feeling part of the emotion is a pattern of sensation in your body. That sensation may be in just one location of your body, but often it fills your whole body. Finally, the urge process typically involves remembering or fantasizing some pleasure associated with the behavior.

The problem is that we only think about the pleasure and forget the far greater pain that the behavior causes. Furthermore, it is important to remember that when you are thinking about the pleasure associated with a behavior, you are also feeling that pleasure in your body. The body pleasure associated with memory and fantasy is sometimes quite subtle and hard to detect. But if you can detect it, you can observe it with detachment. Then it won't turn into a craving. As you can see, the urge process is quite complex. It involves different types of sensations distributed in different spatial patterns throughout your body while at the same time images and conversations are taking place in your mind.

Moreover, all this is constantly changing. The body sensations get strong then weaker. They shift in shape and location. The thoughts speed up then slow down, get louder then softer. Basically the urge process is really nothing more than waves of thought in your mind and sensation in your body. These waves erupt and subside moment by moment. But the phrase 'negative urge' implies something more. It implies a force that drives us to do a behavior which is not in the best interest of ourselves or our loved ones. So there are two key questions that must be answered.

First, how do the thoughts and body sensations turn into this driving force? Second, what should we do about it? Thoughts and body sensations become a driving force when we lock on to them instead of just letting them come and go. By being very attentive, we can break the urge down into its component parts as the urge is happening. We can then watch those individual parts come and go with detachment. The urge then loses much of its force and eventually passes away. Of course it may return again later so we must be ready at all times during the day to detect, observe and stay with the urge until it weakens sufficiently to go on with our lives.

We cannot stop thoughts and feelings from arising, but we can develop the skill of observing them with clarity and detachment until they lose their grip on us. This skill grows with practice, like any other skill. Some people refer to this skill as meditation. It is part of Step 11 in the 12-Step program. Each eruption of the urge represents a new opportunity to strengthen this skill. The urge process consists of a mixture of thoughts and body sensations. You can develop the skill of observing these without locking on to them. To do this you:

- Divide the urge process into its parts.
- Keep track of which parts are present in any given moment.
- Observe the parts in a gentle matter-of-fact way, to the best of your ability.
- Notice how the parts are impermanent, how they rise up and then fade away.

As your skill grows:

- The thoughts and body sensations have less hold over you.
- They pass more quickly and easily.

After long and frequent practice, you may be able to experience the urge as just vibrating energy, like wind through the leaves of a tree or ripples on a still pond.

CHAPTER 16

Shelly's Personal Journey

The earlier description of my Berkeley experience [see page ixx] was a personal account of an utterly desperate and seemingly hopeless individual. What I want you to know is that it has not been an easy journey involving a miraculous, overnight recovery. But with significant perseverance and patience, you too can break out of the sugar prison and be free of all desire for sugar. You can also live a more peaceful and tranquil life.

   I would like to share a personal experience that was very significant in healing my sugar addiction. I attended an intensive mindfulness retreat for several weeks at a time over a period of several months, specifically to work with my sugar addiction. Retreats are very useful because they give you an opportunity for deep changes to take place in a short period of time, since you practice intensively. A retreat also gives you an opportunity to completely face yourself without distraction which helps you get a microscopic look at craving as you learn to apply the methods. My story describes how I applied the mindfulness techniques to my compulsions for sugar. My addiction has not been limited to sugar so I've worked with the methods for all aspects of my addictive behavior. I was not cured of the sugar/food addiction after the retreat, but it helped me see what was possible and gave me a strong foundation for future work. It also cleared away layers of repressed pain from my past. How do I know? This type of knowledge comes from the experience itself and not from intellectual knowledge. Following the retreat, I was never the same as before I went in. It positively and profoundly affected me, not only with my sugar addiction but also with the rest of my life and other suffering issues.

This is my experience and mine alone. It does not mean that your experience will be the same or even similar in regards to working with the discomfort of abstinence from sugar. I will say, however, that in working with any addiction, discomfort has to arise because that's the nature of addiction, even if it is limited to physical withdrawals. If you are driven towards sugar, then you are relieving something uncomfortable by consuming it. If your addiction has an emotional component to it, then you must experience fully, in a mindful way, what the components are as they arise moment to moment. You have possibly destroyed your body and sense of well-being, attempting to avoid feeling. Healing your sugar addiction may be the most challenging endeavor of your life and it will require a consistent and concerted effort on your part.

June 1985 Interview

The following is an interview that was done by a Ph.D. candidate in psychology. The candidate was working on a dissertation regarding significant mindfulness experiences. He requested my participation.

Jim: Shelly, I'd like you to describe in as much detail as possible a particularly powerful or meaningful experience with mindfulness.

Shelly: One of the most powerful experiences for me was attending a two-and-a-half-month meditation retreat last spring in order to get to the bottom of my sugar/food addiction. Prior to the retreat, mindfulness had done much good for me by putting me into a more normal range of eating and helping me to maintain a normal weight. However, I felt ready to go deeper. I wanted to get to the bottom of it and the only way I knew of was to go through the pain within the practice of mindfulness. What that comes down to is having the courage to experience the discomfort fully without indulging in the destructive behavior. This is something that anyone with a sugar/food addiction usually finds impossible to do.

On the retreat, usually by 10 in the morning, cravings were upon me. I would stay with the cravings for eight hours at a time. Until they passed, it was hour after hour of tormenting desire. It was sometimes so intense that I felt that I would surely die from the pain. So at the retreat I had two 17-day stretches like this. For eight hours a day I was in Purgatory. I call it Purgatory because there was a deep healing and purification that took place.

There were many factors that led me to the willingness to stay with this pain in the context of mindfulness practice. Remember, when I say mindful I mean extraordinary attentiveness with an open, non-resistant, radical acceptance of the experience. Even though I was allowing the pain, there was still suffering and it was still difficult. This is because there is an unconscious resistance to it. One must be patient and just accept this until the acceptance penetrates the unconscious.

I reached several breaking points when the pain of craving reached a peak of intensity as my openness to it became greater and greater. Then I would experience tremendous openings where intense emotions would just well up from the depths of my being. I would lie down and do my technique while the pain would well up in my chest which was the major area of emotional blockage for me. I did not know this until I began to practice mindfulness. The methods get you in touch with your body and the blockages created by unconscious holdings. I had some glimpses of this before the retreat, but the retreat situation magnified my thought/feeling process. This is good. It's absolutely necessary to become conscious in order to heal one self.

The first major breakthrough came one day when I felt as though I had to eat sugar. I had to have a sugar binge, and felt as though I couldn't live through the pain of deprivation. There was just no two ways about it. I just had to have sugar! Every addict knows this feeling. But, I didn't do it. First of all, it was difficult to binge on this retreat. That's the power of the retreat situation. It forces you to deal with yourself.

So on this day I decided to give *everything* I had to the mindfulness technique that I was using. It doesn't matter which technique is used. What matters is that you give yourself completely to it. So I literally glued my awareness to the area of my body where I experienced craving. I experienced it as "feel" which was in my chest. It took every bit of willingness and courage to stay with it. I just stayed and stayed and stayed with the technique.

If "talk" or "image" or other sensory experiences pulled my attention away, I would gently return to "feel, I did this even though a huge part of me resisted doing it and was literally screaming, "Eat, eat." As I remained with it, gradually the craving turned into pure feeling. It felt as though my chest was bursting open and this junk was pouring out. And then, finally, it was no longer a craving! It was no longer suffering. I was just pure feelings, old feelings, old pain. It was such a relief. The feelings were absolutely no problem at all.

Jim: What was the pain?

Shelly: Much of the time it was hard to identify the types of feelings. But for the most part they seemed to be old hurt - very old hurt from childhood. Everything felt ancient. There had also been some fear of having a binge. The most important thing to realize, and this is difficult for psychotherapists, is that it doesn't matter what the feelings are or what they mean. All that matters is the mindfulness of them - extraordinary attentiveness and radical acceptance. This is how the deep work on the brain and unconscious occurs.

My experience consisted of a lot of crying and releasing of emotion while in my deepest level of mindfulness. When this was over I felt as though I had experienced a giant orgasm. I was at a much deeper and calmer place within myself.

The following 12 days or so were quite extraordinary. None of the pain that came up ever turned into craving or compulsion.

The feelings that arose just passed through effortlessly. I stayed very mindful in all of my activities and when a hint of craving arose I would open to it and experience its dissolution. For the next few days, the past was literally pouring out of me. It felt like the poison and pain of a lifetime was being released. I had very intense energy rushes. The releasing was absolutely unbelievable! I often had times of eating my meals with absolutely no craving whatsoever. This was quite an unusual experience for me.

After about ten days another level of pain emerged. That's how this process works. You clear out one layer and a deeper layer comes up. Over time, the layers that arise are much easier to handle.

Jim: So the onion always peels deeper.

Shelly: Yes. And the next level was even more intense. I did eat sugar for a week or so, on and off. And then I had another 17-day stretch without sugar. This time the pain was unbearable. Sometimes at the end of the day, I didn't understand how I went through it. I was very grateful for two teachers who were staying there for two weeks. They were very supportive and at least once a day I could talk with either of them. It was the only thing that kept me going. Sometimes I could do nothing but lie in bed and cry. In my entire life I never had the willingness to stay with that kind of discomfort. Part of my willingness came from faith in the mindfulness practice. I had already been through wonderful changes and I knew deep down that this was just the next step to greater freedom. I was correct!

Jim: Give me more details about your second stretch without bingeing.

Shelly: It was unbearable but on a daily basis there were important experiences. The most significant breakthrough came one day after talking to my teacher. I told him that I had decided to leave because I couldn't bear it anymore. So I went back to my room, sat on the floor and was literally beside myself with craving. *Then something happened.* Somehow, in the deepest part of my being, I gave up the struggle against the immense discomfort. One thing is certain - if you stay with the cravings they will always break up and pass away. It is just a matter of time. Impermanence is the nature of everything.

Jim: Thank you, Shelly

CHAPTER 17

Cognitive Behavioral Therapy

Taking an Eclectic Approach to Your Healing

I cannot urge you enough to seek as much support as possible for your healing. Over time, mindfulness leads to permanent changes but in the meantime, you may need support in order to apply mindfulness to your urges for sugar or food. Overeater's Anonymous is one way to go. If you feel adverse to aspects of the program, you can attend with the idea of "take what you like and leave the rest" which is one of their slogans. If nothing else, the phone calls can be very supportive, even if you choose not to go to meetings. There are also telephone and internet meetings available. I have benefited from this program and it continues to influence me in positive ways.

I personally, as well as my clients, have benefited greatly from cognitive-behavioral techniques. I would like to share a particularly powerful technique with you. Cognitive behavioral therapy (CBT) is evidenced-based and shown to be the most effective psychotherapy for food and other addictions. There are many CBT approaches and you can choose one that seems appropriate for you. There are many psychotherapists who specialize in this type of therapy. You can also get self-help books and work on your own. With the method that I am about to describe, you make use of "talk space." When you feel the urge, you begin to create positive, inspiring self-talk. It could be

"I can live without that cookie," or "I'll be so happy if I don't have a binge," or "Being overweight is detrimental to my health."

When the urge comes you bring in the self-talk. Say the words over and over again to yourself. My advice would be to alternate this with the mindfulness method of your choice, so then you are working at a very deep level. What's most important is to stay with your techniques until the urge dissolves or has no hold on you.

In addition to creating positive, inspiring self-talk in the midst of urges, you can make up inspiring 3 x 5 index cards. Write positive, encouraging, inspiring statements on the cards. When you get the urge to eat inappropriately, whip out your cards and read them over and over and over again. You can alternate reading with mindfulness or you can do both at the same time. If you are having strong "feel" then maintain a background awareness of "feel" as you read your cards. Again, stay, stay, stay with it until the urge dissolves or loses its power. The urge will always pass, but you must not try to wish it away. You must leave it alone and allow nature to take its course.

Another helpful hint: if you happen to have strong sugar urges, allow yourself to eat something that you like which is not destructive. This approach can be very helpful. Rome was not built in a day and your sugar problem will not be healed in a day. I personally ate as much as I wanted of healthy foods in order to release sugar. If I got addicted to another food, then I would work with that next.

Eating as much as you want of any healthy food can never be as destructive as bingeing on sugar or refined carbohydrates. I went through and resolved several food addictions, but each served as support for me when that was all I could do. The self-talk that I created at that time was "I'm glad it's this, rather than sugar." This approach takes a strong desire to release perfectionism, which must ultimately be released to free you from sugar addiction. If this is all that you can do, it's better than eating sugar.

I truly wish you the best of luck in this potentially life-transforming endeavor. If you are serious about your desire to break out of the sugar prison, then that amazing freedom can be yours!

CHAPTER 18

Frequently Asked Questions About the Techniques

Q: Is one technique better than another?

A: No. Whatever method you use leads to unconditional freedom. They are all useful for relief of suffering which includes your sugar urges. With all of the methods, you are practicing the skill of mindfulness, which involves concentration, clarity and equanimity.

Q: What should I do if I keep falling asleep?

A: Open your eyes and straighten your posture. If you need to stand up to stay awake, do so. Like any other skill, if you want to learn it, you must be awake and alert. If you want to use the methods at bedtime then you can allow them to help you fall asleep.

Q: What suggestions do you have if I relapse?

A: Notice what arises in your mind/body process at that time. Use a mindfulness method to work with guilt, shame, etc. Anything that arises during relapse will come about as one or more of the basic states described. Apply any technique that you prefer. You can also create constructive self-talk, such as, "It's o.k. I'm not a bad person. I can start again now. It's a new moment." If you follow these instructions it will minimize your suffering around the relapse and reduce its negative impact.

Q: How about internal tunes with or without lyrics? How would you label those?
A: Talk. If you hear internal words then it is always "talk."

Q: How would you label ringing in the ears (tinnitus)?
A: "Sound" since there are no internal words.

Q: How would you label splashes of color?
A: "Blank", since these are no mental pictures.

Q: If it's mostly bright or mostly dark can I label it dark or bright instead of blank?
A: Yes.

Q: How do I label smell or taste?
A: For the sake of convenience, we consider smell or taste to be forms of touch since they are molecules touching the tissues. If you prefer to label them taste and smell, that is fine.

Q: I can't distinguish between the talk and the images.
A: Purposely focus on self-created images, and purposely focus on self-created talk. Take one at a time and this will help you distinguish between them.

Q: I can't distinguish between "feel" and "touch" What should I do?
A: Guess — guessing is perfectly legitimate at any time while you are doing this method. What's most important is that you are making the effort to pay attention to your mind/body process in a gentle, open way. Sooner or later you will know the difference between the states and this can often times be quite useful.

Q: When I'm focusing in image space, all kinds of other things come up at the same time. What should I do?

A: Let those other things be in the background and bring awareness back to "image" or "blank". Nothing is wrong with what arises, and how often it arises. Nothing is wrong with racing thoughts. Nothing is wrong with anything that arises within you because it is nature taking its own natural course. With mindfulness you are not judging nature but rather allowing it to do its own dance within your mind and body. It is only your judgments about it that fool you into believing that it's not perfect just as it is.

Q: Is mindfulness a passive practice? You seem to be talking about doing nothing with your inner experience.

A: I am talking about doing nothing with your mind/body experience. I am talking about getting as close as possible to 100% passivity. However this is *not* an externally passive practice at all! If you can remain internally passive and allow nature to take its course in your own mind and body, then you won't get caught, hooked, trapped, wrapped up in, or controlled by your thoughts, feelings or body experiences. This means, that you will have less or no suffering. In that case, there's a very good probability that you will be able to take actions in the world, in a more efficient, effective, appropriate way. You will not be clouded by unconsciousness. You will be able to think more clearly. You will be able to take actions that you may have been too fearful to engage in.

Here's an example. You're in a theater and there is a fire. Intense "feel" arises and you freeze and panic. You are paralyzed by your experience and sit down on the floor and sob. Your friend has practiced mindfulness. This person can experience feelings without being trapped in them. He allows fear to arise but just lets it be there and even lets it get as big as it wants to get. Even though the fear is big, he is not trapped in it. Therefore it's not controlling his behavior. Without getting trapped in his thoughts or feelings, he immediately walks quickly to the exit and leaves the building. There is potentially a much better outcome for the person who is not overwhelmed by fear.

PART THREE

Learning to Feed Your Body Instead of Your Addiction

CHAPTER 19

The Sugar Prison Diet

The Sugar Prison Diet is a perfect, daily, dietary companion that can accommodate all of your nutritional needs. It is divided into two easy steps. There are two optional segments to each step. In other words, you can mix and match as you see fit. You are free to maintain control of the dietary segment of this protocol from start to finish.

Step One:

Option A: 7-day therapeutic fast, also known as a liquid diet. It allows your body to rest, rejuvenate nerve force, throw off toxic waste and begin the cellular rebuilding and replacement process.

Option B: 21-day transitional diet. This allows you to accomplish most of what will take place during the fast but at a slower pace.

Step Two:

Option A: 30-day sample menu. Learn how to intelligently plan nutritious meals to continue the cellular rejuvenation and rebuilding process you initiated during Step One.

Option B: A quick and simple daily menu for busy sugar addicts. Intended for use if your schedule is too hectic to follow the entire nutritional program recommended above.

I recommend that you begin with the 7-day therapeutic fast. If you are diabetic, hypoglycemic or suffer from some other serious metabolic, emotional or psychological disorder, it may be wiser for you to consider going through the 21-day transitional diet instead of the therapeutic fast. If you have questions regarding the safety or advisability of going through the fast or transitional diet, you should consult with a knowledgeable health practitioner beforehand.

The 21-day transitional diet, although not as powerful in its deep-tissue cleansing action as the therapeutic fast, can help jump-start the process of reversing any addictive tendencies you may have to refined carbohydrates. After completing the fast or 21-day diet, please proceed to Step Two. The daily menus recommended there will help strengthen and rebuild your body.

Getting the Best Results from a Therapeutic Fast or 21-Day Transitional Diet

I usually recommend that anyone at the beginning stages of reversing sugar addiction clean out the body's waste elimination channels as thoroughly as possible. Depending on the case, I would suggest a series of four colon irrigations or high enemas with no more than three days between each session. The first two sessions should be done on consecutive days. Colonics or high enemas can help establish a clean base of operations so nature can start correcting your physiological dysfunction with the least degree of difficulty.

Even if you do not choose to take this preliminary step, here are additional suggestions to help you achieve optimal results from either doing a fast or following the transitional diet.

- ♦ Stop consuming junk beverages and foods - especially starchy carbohydrates - prior to and immediately following the fast or the 21-day diet. They will only exacerbate your existing condition.

- Stop doing whatever activities tend to drain your energy on a daily basis – emotional, mental or unnecessary physical activity can be a needless drag on the very nerve force your body is in need of now.

- Start making an effort to get sufficient rest every day, especially during this entire program. Your body cannot effectively heal itself of disease or replace distressed and worn out tissue unless you allow it to rest daily.

- If you decide to do the fast, after you successfully complete it, you must start consuming whole foods and beverages that can quickly rebuild and replace formerly weak and distressed tissue.

- If you do the initial therapeutic fast, you may want to consider a follow-up fast of five to seven days in four months, and a third fast of five days in eight months for best results.

- When you take a shower, start with warm water and then let a cool spray hit your entire body during the final minute of the shower. This will help circulation – particularly to the interior organs, nerves and other tissues. **Special Note**: DO NOT use a cool spray on your body if you feel excessively feeble or suffer with high blood pressure or a weak heart condition.

- Whichever method you choose, engage in some form of exercise daily to ensure muscle tone, proper elimination of bodily waste, and good blood and lymph flow. Massage, Tai Chi, brisk walking, swimming, Shiatsu and other physically stimulating routines can be useful.

- Each day, do the various mindfulness exercises recommended in Part Two. Your attitude and outlook now are critical elements for success.

- Use the *Weekly Diet and Nutrition Worksheets* and the *Daily Mindfulness for Life Worksheets* in the Appendix to keep a written record of your mental, emotional and physiological experiences, beginning with the first day of the therapeutic fast or the 21-day diet.

Optional but recommended

- Begin getting at least one half hour of direct sunshine daily. This will help increase your vitality, nerve force and will ensure the natural production of vitamin D which is essential for control and assimilation of organic calcium in your body. **Special Note**: DO NOT expose yourself to direct sunlight if you have skin cancer or some other sunlight-sensitive health condition.
- Begin to practice five or ten minutes of deep breathing exercises daily – this will also help rebuild nerve force and more efficiently clean carbon dioxide out of the blood stream.
- Begin brushing your skin for three minutes on a daily basis prior to taking a shower. Use a natural bristle medium tension brush. This will open the pores, help get rid of uric acid crystals in the pores and on the skin and aid the kidneys, lungs and colon in ridding your body of toxic waste.

If you have any serious questions or concerns about the nutritional aspect of this protocol, I invite you to contact me at our website; breakoutofthesugarprison.com. Let's be sure you are staying on the right track to wellness.

CHAPTER 20

Letting Nature Cleanse, Rest and Rejuvenate Your Body

Step One/Option A

The Powerful Secret of Why a Fast Can Help You Quickly Overcome Your Sugar Addiction

Nature has endowed your body with an amazing mechanism that can greatly enhance your efforts to overcome sugar addiction – a simple but powerful process known as autolysis.

What exactly is autolysis? The following analogy might explain it best: Imagine buying a fixer-upper old house in need of a lot of repairs. What is the first thing you do after a home inspector tells you about all of the things you will need to do to bring the house up to code and make it a safe and habitable place?

You clean it out and scrub it down to see what you really have to work with, right? You need to see what is left of the house - the bare bones so to speak. This way you will know what you need to do to get the house the way you want it.

You start scrubbing the walls, ceiling and floors, cleaning out any congested plumbing pipes, and tearing out old material wherever necessary, as you prepare the house for the new materials you plan to replace the old.

This is similar to what your body goes through during autolysis. Autolysis is a process that kicks into gear when your body has been on a liquid diet, or fast, for about three days. Beginning with the third or fourth day, your body senses it needs to find more nutriment than what it is being fed from the juices, teas and broth you have been drinking. Your body must, after all, continue to feed all of your cells – especially the brain, heart and central nervous system.

Here is where nature's mysterious power of autolysis comes into play. While your body is on the fast, it will break down fatty deposits, toxins and drugs, thick deposits of mucus, cysts, tumors, excess skin accumulations and non-essential bodily fluids. It does not do this because it wants you to be healthy and well, per se. Your body will do this out of its nature-driven need to supply its cells with a constant source of nutrients.

Once the process of autolysis kicks in, your body will continue this general housecleaning until it completely throws away any carbon-bearing, fermented material it is able to dislodge and remove through defecation, urination, sweating, spitting and breathing. This deep-tissue cleansing process can go on for a couple of weeks or even a month or two, depending on the person and the length of the fast.

It will usually continue until your body's nutritional reserves begin to run low. At that point your body will develop a natural hunger for food that a glass or two of raw juice, tea, broth or water will not satisfy. This is nature's signal that your body is ready to start eating food again.

The ideal length of time to allow autolysis to run its course is at least three weeks for most biological disorders. However, I have found that, in cases of sugar or other substance abuse correction, 7 to 14 days is sufficient to get the healing ball rolling.

This is the main reason for my insistence that you stop chasing after herbal preparations, space-age food supplements and health drinks until your body is in a position to take advantage of them. None of these things can do you any lasting good unless you first allow your entire body to rest, cleanse itself, rejuvenate your vital force and then start rebuilding along healthy lines.

One of the nicest things to hear is a patient talking about how wonderful and rejuvenated she feels after autolysis has run its course. I have had people tearfully thank me for giving them back their bodies and their lives when, actually, I was only a small spark that fueled the fire of their drive and determination to reclaim their health.

This was their show. I was only a concerned spectator. And the first major step in doing this was inviting the autolysis process to work its magic. There is nothing like having a clean, strong and responsive body handed back to you on nature's silver platter.

Basic Elements of the Therapeutic Fast

Following are instructions for preparing juices you will need to utilize during the therapeutic fast. Start with a good juicer. Then, you'll need to have the following items on hand on a daily basis:

- 20 raw carrots
- 5 stalks of raw celery
- 1 raw white turnip
- 1 raw red beet
- 1 raw cucumber
- 1 raw sweet potato
- 3 sprigs raw parsley

Through trial and error, I have found these seven raw vegetables to have a high concentration of wonderful biochemical elements your body can use to good advantage while you are fasting. These elements will, for the most part, bypass the digestive processes of the stomach and small intestine and be absorbed directly into your blood stream.

You will want to prepare your juice each morning or evening as follows:

Juice the raw vegetables together, let stand for five minutes and strain. Discard the hardened starchy residue and keep the juice. Mix two parts juice with one part room-temperature distilled or other purified water and drink a glass slowly. Refrigerate the remaining juice immediately.

The juice will retain close to full potency for a few hours. After that it will lose some nutritional value with each passing hour that it is kept refrigerated or transported in a thermos. Consume within 36 to 48 hours maximum but within 24 hours is optimal. If you are unable to make the juice at home, locate a health food store that can prepare what you need.

It is important that you not eat anything or take any food supplements during the entire seven-day therapeutic fast. If you are currently on prescribed medication, you should consult with your doctor to determine if it would be possible for you to engage the fast without taking all or some of your medication. If at all possible, it is best to undertake the fast with only the juices, broth and water recommended in this protocol. You must allow nature an opportunity to do what she can to correct any physiological dysfunction as best she can. Nature can only do this if you allow her natural cleansing process of autolysis to take place.

Step-By-Step Guide for Conducting and Finishing the 7-Day Therapeutic Fast

During waking hours, drink a 10 to 12-ounce glass of raw vegetable juice every 2 hours, every day of the 7-day fast. If the raw, undiluted juice seems thick or has a taste that is too strong or bitter, you can dilute it with purified water. Mix 2 parts raw juice with 1 part water and drink. You should not experience acute hunger if you follow this schedule. If you should feel hungry, drink more juice or purified water whenever necessary.

Another vital part of this fasting program is to have a cup of cooked vegetable broth 2 or 3 hours before bedtime. This highly alkaline broth can help reduce the incidence of occasional pain and discomfort while on the fast. (The recipe for my healthy alkaline vegetable broth can be found in the Appendix)

The Proper Way to Break Your Fast

How you go about breaking your fast is as important as the fast itself. During the fast your digestive juices almost completely stop flowing into the stomach and small intestines and the muscles of the large bowel tend to go to sleep. Fasting is a resting period for most of the body. Your body slows down the functions of whatever organs and systems are not considered vital to keeping it alive.

The first day you decide to break your fast, the first few meals should be light and easy to digest and assimilate. For example, I suggest you begin eating a small green, leafy salad without dressing at lunch on the first day of food - the eighth day of the fast. The salad is the only solid food you should have on that day, along with the recommended liquids you have been taking during your fast.

On the ninth and tenth days continue with the raw juices and vegetable broth and the same small, raw salad plus an unpeeled baked potato or a bowl of brown rice for lunch.

When you decide to break your fast, the functions of your stomach, liver and intestines must be jump-started slowly so that they can be gradually brought back to full operation. You want to do this without overburdening these organs with large, heavy meals that cannot be processed efficiently immediately following your fast.

After the therapeutic fast and the subsequent three-day fast-breaking periods are over you can start eating nutritionally balanced, healthy meals. You'll find dozens of tasty and nutritious recipes later in this book.

Step One/Option B

21-Day Transitional Diet

(Use this diet in place of the therapeutic fast for moderate but steady results)

The primary goal of this 21-day transitional diet is to slowly and intelligently prepare your body for an overhaul of all its glands, organs and systems. You will be focusing on correcting any dysfunction in your adrenals, pancreas, liver, your entire endocrine organization, and all other bodily systems. Although such a process can take months to successfully accomplish, you must begin somewhere.

You will be transitioning to a healthier way to eat and live as you eliminate old, stagnant, unhealthy tissue in exchange for tissue that is vibrantly healthy and functional. In the process, your blood sugar level should stabilize within a healthy range. Provided that you simultaneously practice the appropriate daily mindfulness exercises, you should begin to lose your unhealthy addiction to or unhealthy desire for, sugar and starchy carbohydrates, within a reasonably short time – perhaps a month or two.

The components of the 21-day transitional diet are certain ripe fruit, fruit juice, raw and steamed vegetables, vegetable broth and high quality protein. If possible, it's preferable to use organic cottage cheese, kefir, yogurt, goat whey, raw tahini, raw sunflower seeds, whole grain rye products, almonds, soy milk powder, brown rice protein powder, cow whey or other high-quality proteins during this time.

Before you get started, there are a few things to be aware of that you *should not do*:

- ♦ Do not drink any alcoholic beverages, coffee, sodas, artificially flavored drinks or tap water during this 21-day period.

- Do not consume any strong spices.
- Do not smoke or chew any tobacco products.
- Do not eat anything made with processed sugar or denatured flour.
- Do not use a lot of salt with food – excess salt consumption can cause a loss of potassium which can contribute to low blood sugar.

As for the things you *should* do:

- Each day, engage in some form of exercise that utilizes your legs, arms and torso.
- Take a warm shower or relaxing bath each evening before bedtime, when possible. If you're carrying a lot of excess water weight, skip this suggestion.
- Practice the daily affirmations and other suggestions given to you in the mindfulness section of this program. They will help you make the whole-being transition to wellness much more complete and satisfying.
- Get plenty of rest each day.

21-Day Menu

Breakfast

- When you awaken, stir two tablespoons of liquid chlorophyll or wheat grass juice into five ounces of purified, room-temperature water. Drink with two kelp supplements. Do not eat anything for at least 30 minutes.
- For breakfast, alternate the following three options at your discretion:

Option #1 (Best choice) - Drink a 12-ounce glass of my whole foods blended cocktail. (See recipe in the Appendix). If desired, you can also have a slice of whole grain rye or sprouted rye bread toast with organic butter or a tablespoon of raw wheat germ. Drink *slowly* and chew *thoroughly*! (I highly recommend this option. It has been my favorite breakfast for two decades).

Option #2 - Eat an 8 ounce serving of plain, organic cottage cheese, yogurt or kefir or an animal protein of your choice. Include half a grapefruit or an eight ounce serving of strawberries and blueberries. If you drink any fluid, limit it to no more than six ounces of herbal tea, purified water or grapefruit juice.

Option #3 - Eat a single serving of cooked whole grain cereal high in silicon, such as oats, barley, rye or brown rice. You can have a slice or two of whole grain, sprouted rye bread with organic butter. If you drink any fluid, limit it to no more than six ounces of herbal tea, raw vegetable juice or purified water.

Supplements to take with options #2 or #3 (Preferably, you should take as many of these as possible in powdered or liquid form):

- Multivitamin
- One teaspoon of bee pollen or a single serving of royal jelly
- Two tablespoons of real brewer's yeast
- 10 chlorella tablets or capsules (200 mgs each)
- Multi-mineral supplement with manganese and chromium
- Lecithin
- Digestive aid with HCL and pepsin. (If you can't find this, a good, natural substitute I use is one half tablespoon of organic apple cider vinegar)

Mid-morning snack

Eat half a ripe grapefruit or have some other ripe fruit that you do not have a tendency to binge on. You can also have a handful of raw almonds or raw sunflower seeds.

Lunch

Option #1 - Eat a large raw salad with the following vegetables; romaine or red leaf lettuce, cucumber, alfalfa sprouts, celery, cauliflower and tomatoes. For dressing, use a tablespoon of seed oil or pure and cold pressed virgin olive oil and a pinch of organic sea salt. You can have one or two slices of whole grain or sprouted rye bread or a few rye crackers with a small amount of organic butter, if desired. If you drink any fluid, limit it to no more than six ounces of raw vegetable juice, herbal tea or purified water.

Option #2 - Eat a handful of raw sunflower seeds, raw tahini (sesame) or raw almonds along with grapefruit, apples, papaya, strawberries or blueberries. You can also have plain, organic cottage cheese, kefir or yogurt with a half or whole grapefruit for lunch. If you drink any fluid, limit it to no more than six ounces of raw fruit juice, herbal tea or purified water.

Supplements to take with either option:

- Multivitamin
- One teaspoon of bee pollen or a single serving of royal jelly
- Two tablespoons of brewer's yeast
- 10 chlorella tablets or capsules (200 mgs each)
- Multi-mineral supplement with manganese and chromium
- Lecithin
- Digestive aid with HCL and pepsin.

Mid-afternoon snack

Raw fruit, strawberries or blueberries with yogurt, kefir or cottage cheese and grapefruit juice with raw nuts or seeds, are good snack combinations.

Dinner

Steamed or lightly cooked vegetables, baked potato with jacket or a bowl of brown rice or brown and wild rice. You can have a raw vegetable salad with a tablespoon of cold pressed virgin olive oil and a pinch sea salt or a teaspoon of organic apple cider vinegar for dressing, if you desire. A small serving of protein from the breakfast menu earlier in the day is okay or you may prefer a serving of cooked beans or lentil soup. You can have one slice of whole grain rye or sprouted rye bread or rye crackers. Have no more than 6 ounces of herbal tea or purified water with this meal.

Supplements:

- Multivitamin
- Multi-mineral supplement with manganese and chromium
- Digestive aid with HCL and pepsin.

Mid-evening

Have a warm cup of unsweetened chamomile and dandelion tea or a cup of alkaline vegetable broth, if desired. (See recipe for alkaline vegetable broth in Appendix). Eat nothing solid.

Bedtime

If you are tired but unable to sleep, take four tablets of the homeopathic cell salt calcium phosphate, along with a strong cup of unsweetened dandelion and chamomile tea. This should help you drift into a restful sleep. (A warm cup of valerian or other sleep-inducing herbal tea can be used instead).

LETTING NATURE CLEANSE, REST & REJUVENATE YOUR BODY

While you are following this diet, it is important that you get plenty of sleep, sunshine, exercise requiring a reasonable degree of strength and endurance and breathe fresh air as often as possible. This will help revitalize your nerve force (your body's electrical power) and help your glands, organs and systems function more efficiently.

Among other benefits, this program can help stabilize your blood sugar level, regulate your weight, give you more energy and help you establish a restful sleep pattern. You should start this program soon, while it is fresh in your mind and your enthusiasm is high.

When you have completed the 21-day transitional diet, proceed to Step Two – Wholesome and Healthy Maintenance Menus. Remember to make a written note in the *Weekly Diet and Nutrition Worksheets* and the *Daily Mindfulness for Life Worksheets*, of your mental, emotional and physiological experiences while on the therapeutic fast or the 21-day transitional diet. Both can be found in the Appendix.

CHAPTER 21

Wholesome and Healthy Maintenance Menus

Step Two/Option A

A 30-Day Sample Menu to Use after You Break Your Fast or Complete the 21-Day Transitional Diet

This entire program is designed to slowly but surely clean, rejuvenate and rebuild your sugar-whipped, abused body. It takes time, but you *will* get there.

You should be able to kick your habit and desire for sugar and other harmful carbohydrate products within a month or two. However, it can take three or four months, or even a year, before your body will show significant improvement in your overall health depending on the rate your body replaces old, worn out, distressed cellular tissue with vibrantly healthy new tissue.

Recovery time is also dependent on your ability to develop and maintain a healthy bloodstream. You must have a good, ample supply of red blood cells to attract oxygen to the body and, of course, sufficient reserves of sodium phosphate to remove carbon dioxide and other waste from your cells and bloodstream.

Oxygen enters your body through your pores, and while ingesting food and drink. However, your main concern should be the amount of oxygen entering your body through your bloodstream which subsequently transports it to each cell of your body to carry out cellular metabolism.

Cellular metabolism is simply the process where the food you eat is transformed or chemically burned in each cell and made ready for heat or energy production, or for building and restoring bodily tissue.

The residue created in each cell by the food that is processed, and by the breakdown of cellular tissue that is being replaced by new tissue, is continuously being transported back into the bloodstream, lymph or intercellular fluid. The waste material is then eliminated from your body – at least under ideal circumstances.

The key is to have as smooth an operation as possible to ensure your entire body is being fed its necessary, daily allotment of fuel and that the toxic garbage which ordinarily accumulates with each passing moment is being evacuated as often as necessary. Both of these important processes - anabolism and catabolism - must function in an efficient, timely manner to ensure your health and well-being.

You can see how sugar addiction can make it hard for these two important metabolic processes to take place without difficulty. The more sugar you ingest, the greater the carbon buildup in your tissues and the greater the need for oxygen and sodium phosphate, the harder you make it for your body to carry out basic, vitally important functions at the cellular level.

The therapeutic fast or 21-day transitional diet, combined with one of the two follow-up 30-day menus, can afford you a priceless opportunity to properly regulate your metabolic rate. When it comes to reversing the bad effects of sugar abuse and addiction on your body, a properly functioning metabolism is worth its weight in platinum.

The following sample of a healthy, daily meals menu can help your body stabilize your metabolic rate naturally and intelligently. Keep in mind the necessity for variety and regularity in eating and drinking wholesome foods and beverages. Your body will mold to whatever it's fed – either to coffee and doughnuts, or to good, wholesome meals. The choice is yours.

Bear in mind this is only a sample of the kind of meals you may want to prepare for yourself following the therapeutic fast. Specific menus you can enjoy appear in the Appendix. Use your imagination to come up with a routine that includes variety, tasty dishes and nutritious preparations pleasing to all your senses.

If you have a difficult time deciding what you should prepare at any time following your fast and fast breaking periods, contact me and together you and I will come up with something sensible and easy for you to follow.

If you are diabetic or hypoglycemic, consult with a nutritionally knowledgeable health practitioner before preparing any of the dishes or using any of the natural sweets mentioned in the menu choices.

30-Day Sample Menu

Breakfast

- 30 minutes prior to breakfast, mix one tablespoon of pure black cherry concentrate or liquid chlorophyll with six ounces of silicon tonic and drink slowly (Recipe for silicon tonic is in the Appendix).
- For breakfast, alternate the following three options at your discretion

Option A: Have the whole foods blended cocktail with whole grain rye bread or crackers. Add a little organic butter and raw honey if desired. **Caution**: Do not use honey if you feel it will trigger an urge to binge.

Option B: Have cold whole grain cereal with almond and sesame nut milk. Sprinkle on raw oats, raw sunflower seeds, a little raw wheat germ and ground up flaxseeds.

Option C: If you like dairy, consider having a bowl of organic yogurt or cottage cheese, ripe strawberries and blueberries or apple slices and a piece of whole grain bread, lightly toasted.

Supplements:

- Multivitamin
- Chlorella tablets or capsules - 200 mgs each (10)
- Multi-mineral with manganese and chromium
- Lecithin – 1 serving size
- Digestive aid with HCL and pepsin
- Kelp – 3 tablets or one half teaspoon of granules or powder

Mid-morning

Option A: Black cherry juice, grapefruit juice, apple juice, papaya nectar, herbal tea, purified water or have a glass of nut and seed milk.

Option B: Eat a serving of acid or sub-acid fruit, such as citrus, apple, peach, pear or papaya with a handful of raw nuts and/or seeds – be sure to chew thoroughly.

Lunch

Option A: Tossed green salad with avocado, sprouts, tomato, cucumber and a cold-pressed vegetable oil or cream dressing. Have a serving of whole grain crackers or whole grain or sprouted grain bread with a little organic sweet butter if desired. Have a small glass of purified water or a cup of herbal tea or a little lemon juice squeezed into a small glass of water.

Option B: Have Swiss or hard cheddar cheese or organic cottage cheese and apple slices, strawberries or blueberries.

Option C: Have organic unsweetened yogurt with raw nuts and raw fruit.

Supplements:

- Multivitamin
- Chlorella tablets or capsules - 200 mgs each (10)
- Multi-mineral supplement with manganese and chromium
- Lecithin – 1 serving size
- Digestive aid with HCL and pepsin
- Kelp – 3 tablets or one half teaspoon of granules or powder

Mid-afternoon

Option A: Black cherry juice, grapefruit juice, apple juice, papaya nectar, herbal tea, purified water or have a glass of nut and seed milk.

Option B: Eat a serving of acid or sub-acid fruit, such as citrus, apple, peach, pear or papaya with a handful of raw nuts and/or seeds – be sure to chew thoroughly

Dinner

Select any combination of the following:

- Steamed vegetables, light serving of your preferred protein, baked, unpeeled, sweet or russet potato.
- Any homemade healthy soup.
- Steamed vegetables.
- Slice or two of whole grain, sprouted bread.
- Small green salad if desired.
- Brown rice or whole grain pasta.

- Vegetable juice or peppermint and dandelion tea or purified water.

Mid-evening

Drink a cup of dandelion tea, peppermint tea or vegetable broth. Eat nothing solid within three hours of bedtime. Take a warm bath or shower before having your tea or broth, if desired. It will help settle your nerves and prepare you for a good night's rest.

Bedtime

If you are awake and thirsty, drink a cup of some soothing herbal tea, such as chamomile and dandelion tea or have a small cup of silicon tonic or a small glass of purified, tepid water.

Although the indication is for a 30-day dietary, I strongly suggest that you follow the above sample menu as closely as possible for at least three months for best results. This may seem like a lot to do but, I give you my word that this can help you tremendously.

During this 30-day sample menu, I advise that you consume no more than 2 or 3 ounces of high-quality protein daily. Try not to exceed this amount; however, any less can put you at risk for a drop in sustained energy levels throughout the day. As a protein source, consider raw nut and seed milks, organic cottage cheese, soy milk and soybeans, brewer's yeast, lentils, sweet peas, whole grain rye, quinoa, kefir, yogurt, raw almond butter, raw organic goat milk, raw sunflower seeds or butter, raw tahini and sesame seeds, tofu and various high-quality animal proteins of your choosing.

Try to keep your intake of animal flesh products to a minimum during any meal where you have vegetable oil on salad or otherwise with the meal. The oil will slow down the digestion of protein in the stomach and small intestine. Much of the protein will pass undigested down to the large bowel where it will meet with the lactobacilli bacteria and begin to putrefy. In the

Appendix you will find a number of tasty, high protein sample recipes that can satisfy your body's daily protein requirements.

To assist with the breakdown of excess, harmful carbon waste products and mucus within your body, you should have one or more of the following foods daily. They are all high in formic acid:

- Apples
- Dwarf nettles tea or powder
- Florida or California organic oranges
- Grapefruit
- Lemons
- Limes
- Pine needle broth or tea, or add ground pine needles to raw vegetable salads
- Tangerines

When combined with the cell salt sodium phosphate (natrum phos.), organic formic acid can effectively and safely help reduce the fermenting tendency of excess, unorganized sugar throughout your body.

Included with your meals are food items high in the trace element chromium. Chromium is a major player involved with blood sugar control. It combines in the blood with insulin in such a way that your cell walls can allow glucose to pass through without difficulty. The lower the amount of chromium present in your blood stream, the less effective your body will be in feeding energy- and heat-producing sugar molecules to each cell. Consequently, chronic chromium deficiency can contribute to the development of diabetes mellitus and other sugar-related abnormalities.

The biochemical element manganese has an affinity for the brain, nerves, cartilage and ligaments. Many of the carbon-related aches and pains you may feel from time to time can have their roots in a manganese deficiency. It has also been proven to be helpful for blood sugar control. I've included foods that are high in manganese in the above 30-day sample menu.

In the event you feel that, for whatever reasons, you cannot follow the therapeutic fast or the 21-day transitional diet, or even the 30-day sample menu, I suggest you try my quick and simple daily menu for busy sugar addicts. I am not advocating that you forego the preliminary steps to completely overcoming your sugar addiction, but I am aware of the realities of everyday life. There are days when you cannot find time or motivation to do what you know to be the right thing. But I hope you will go through the preliminary stages. The protocol is designed in such a way that one phase of it naturally and intelligently flows into the next. That is how it should be in an ideal world. Be that as it may, I would rather you do something right rather than nothing at all.

Step Two/Option B

Quick and Simple Daily Menu for Busy Sugar Addicts

If your busy professional, academic or homemaker schedule will not afford you the luxury of following the fast, 21 day diet or 30 day sample menu, this should fit you like a glove. It's a bit more streamlined than the 30 day sample menu, easier to follow and you can derive great benefit by adhering to it. In case you are wondering, for the past two decades, *this is the daily menu I have tended to follow*. I usually have the whole foods blended drink once daily - with or as my breakfast.

Food items: Ideally, every day, divided between *all* of your meals, have the following:

- 6 low-starch, raw salad vegetables
- 1 or 2 steamed or lightly cooked vegetables

WHOLSOME AND HEALTHY MAINTENANCE MENUS

- 2 pieces of raw fruit or a serving of ripe strawberries or blueberries
- 1 major starch (such as bread, potatoes or corn)
- 1 major serving of a protein of your choice (try not to mix starchy vegetables or whole grain products with large servings of protein or with citrus fruit or fruit drinks at the same meal).

Between meal snacks and beverages: Fruit, berries, raw nuts and seeds. When preferred, have a glass of fruit juice, nut and seed milk (see recipe in Appendix), raw vegetable juice or purified water. Drink peppermint, chamomile or dandelion tea at night, if desired.

Supplements: With breakfast and lunch, take the following (preferably, you should take as many of these as possible in powdered or liquid form or in a blended drink):

- Multivitamin
- Chlorella tablets or capsules - 200 mgs each (10)
- Multi-mineral supplement with manganese and chromium
- Lecithin – 1 serving size
- Digestive aid with HCL and pepsin
- Kelp – 3 tablets or one half teaspoon of granules

At least 4 days each week, drink 8 to10 ounces of my whole foods blended cocktail with or as your breakfast. (See recipe in Appendix). Eat nothing solid within 3 hours of bedtime.

It may be easier for you to take the supplements as part of a healthy blended cocktail each day. Breakfast is my preferred time for drinking my whole foods blended cocktail. If you are not allergic to *bee pollen, brewer's yeast* or raw and organic *apple cider vinegar*, I highly recommend that you include a teaspoon of bee pollen, one tablespoon of apple cider vinegar and two tablespoons of brewer's yeast in your health cocktail.

If you develop flatulence, omit the brewer's yeast for a day to see if that is the culprit. If so, omit entirely from the menu for two weeks. Try taking one tablespoon daily of brewer's yeast beginning the third week. Work your way back up to three to four tablespoons daily if possible. There is an excellent reason why I am asking you to do this. The combination of kelp, bee pollen, apple cider vinegar, chlorella, soya lecithin and brewer's yeast can have a profoundly beneficial effect on your health and energy level.

Friendly Reminder: If you have not begun completing the *Weekly Diet and Nutrition Worksheets* and the *Daily Mindfulness for Life Worksheet* that accompany this protocol, please take the time now to begin doing so. You will find these forms in the Appendix. They should not consume too much of your time each day and can prove valuable as a reference tool.

Healthy Food Items You can Consume after the Fast or 21-Day Transitional Diet

Below is a listing of items that can give you the extra boost you may need to add zip to your step and support your body with wonderful combinations of biochemical elements. You can begin adding these to your diet once you start the 30-day sample menu or the quick and simple daily menu for busy sugar addicts.

- Alfalfa sprouts
- Blue green algae
- Brewer's yeast
- Brown and wild rice
- Buckwheat flour
- Celery
- Clabbered or fermented foods made from raw organic milk
- Cold-pressed, unheated seed and nut oils

- Dulse
- Garlic
- Goat whey
- Hawthorne berry tea or tincture
- Homeopathic cell salts
- Kelp
- Lettuce
- Most raw fruits in season
- Most raw seeds
- Most raw vegetables
- Most whole grains
- MSM
- Oats, oat water and oat straw tea
- Onions
- Organic apple cider vinegar (use sparingly)
- Prunes
- Raw black walnuts
- Raw organic milk (preferably goat milk)
- Raw wheat germ
- Red clover tea or tincture
- Royal jelly
- Silicon water extracted from raw oats, barley and wheat bran
- Soya lecithin
- Spirulina
- Wheat bran water or tea
- Wheat grass juice

You should never hesitate to take supplements derived from whole foods and herbs whenever you suspect your foods are not providing you with a wide assortment of the necessary nutrients your body must have in order to ensure efficient metabolic and physiological function. There may come a time when you will have no need to take another supplement again.

However, if you are uncertain about the nutritive quality of your foods, then by all means continue taking supplements to augment the nutritive content of your foods and beverages.

Stay Away from or Minimize Your Use of These Denatured Foods and Beverages

How you end the dietary portion of the entire protocol is every bit as important as how it is begun. You can undo a month or two of wonderful cleansing and cellular rejuvenation activity with one poorly conceived meal. Be sure to steer clear of these health-destroying foods and beverages for at least three months after beginning this protocol.

- Processed wheat products
- Refined sugar products
- Processed honey, molasses, jellies or syrups
- Alcohol
- Smoking or chewing tobacco
- Black caffeinated tea
- Coffee
- Black pepper
- Table salt
- Strong spices of any kind
- Candy
- White or distilled vinegar
- Pasteurized milk and its by-products
- Commercially prepared pies and cakes
- Toasted or salted nuts or seeds
- Unripe or excessively over-ripe fruit of any kind

Basic Laws of Eating

Here are a handful of suggestions that can help you reap a harvest of health and wellness that could last 100 years or more.

- Eat a full meal only when you are really hungry – not whenever you have an appetite
- Eat until you are no longer hungry but not quite full
- Chew your food reasonably well to ensure good digestive action
- Do not eat anything solid if you are upset, excited or feeling sick
- Use light vegetable or seed oils for occasional frying
- At least 80% of your daily intake of food should be alkaline
- At least 65 to 75% of your daily food intake should be raw and uncooked
- Have a raw salad at least five days weekly using no less than five different vegetables as part of your long-term health maintenance strategy
- Try not to drink anything very hot or icy cold with meals
- Eat some type of natural, whole grain food product daily
- Try not to drink more than six ounces of any fluid with any given meal
- Eat moderately so you do not overwork the liver, adrenals, gall bladder and pancreas
- Drink purified water instead of tap water
- Never use any kind of aluminum cookware
- Do not drink citrus fruit juice when experiencing inflammations

- Your heaviest meal should be eaten at lunchtime. That is when your digestive system will usually be working at maximum efficiency
- The later in the day you eat, the less protein you should have
- Do not mix citrus fruit with heavy starches
- When you serve a meal with a large percentage of protein, be sure to limit the amount of heavy starches during that same meal

The key here is to not be fanatical. Exercise reason and good judgment as you keep the above suggestions in mind. Enjoy your meals and your life.

CHAPTER 22

Start NOW to Break Out of the Sugar Prison

Welcome to the first day of the rest of your healthy life. Both of us are confident you will stretch even farther than what you think you can, to start breaking out of the sugar prison. Here's a recap of what we're encouraging you to do.

- Start the therapeutic fast or 21-day transitional diet – along with your daily mindfulness exercises. When you have finished the fast or transitional diet, start either the 30-day sample menu or the quick and simple daily menu for busy sugar addicts.

- Resolve to do whatever it takes to get your life back on track and reclaim your health and happiness.

- Forget about rereading every line and word in this book, hoping you will uncover an effortless way to break your shackles and free yourself from the sugar prison without personal effort. It is not going to happen that way. Get going *now* and do something constructive to turn your life around. Get started with the protocol outlined in this book, *today*!

Conclusion

Uprooting destructive tendencies is one of the greatest challenges a human being can undertake. Ultimately, you are dealing with the issue of dissatisfaction and the seeking of peacefulness outside of yourself. This incessant longing is not just the story of your addictive behaviors, but the story of your life and the lives of others. When you decide to break the shackles of addictive tendencies - whether with sugar or other aspects of your life - you will find that, at the deepest level of your being, the tendency to grasp pleasure and reject discomfort is at the root of all discontent.

You alone must first access the inherent strength and power within you that will allow you to move forward at a steady pace. No one can do this for you. However, we can point you in a constructive direction and help you build the kind of momentum that can lead to meaningful change. Sometimes it takes a dramatic and rather painful "hitting bottom." Hopefully you can avoid the immense suffering involved with that. However, there are times when that is exactly what is required. It can be exactly what you need to experience significant and lasting change. We, the authors, have lived this bottom. It was what we needed to turn our lives around.

We are pleased that you have taken the time to read and digest the wealth of information regarding our powerful mindfulness and nutritional systems. It has been a great joy to share our experience and knowledge with you.

If you should have any questions or concerns about the protocol, or if at any point along the road to recovery and reclamation of your life you feel you could use a little encouragement, contact Paul about any aspect of the nutritional component of the protocol or Shelly about mindfulness issues.

May you experience great and lasting success on your healing journey.

Appendix

Worksheets

Daily Mindfulness for Life
Weekly Diet and Nutrition

Please complete a *Daily Mindfulness for Life Worksheet* and *Weekly Diet and Nutrition Worksheet* for the entire protocol. We have found it to be more advantageous to make daily entries rather than waiting to the end of a given week to complete the Diet and Nutrition worksheets. For your convenience we have numbered the Diet and Nutrition worksheets as weeks one through seven. Complete the information requested on each week's worksheet to the best of your ability. On the mindfulness worksheet you can make useful notes and reading the sheet daily can serve as a helpful reminder of potential challenges to watch for.

You may have questions and concerns during the course of this program. If you would like for one of us to review and comment on a given week's activities for you, use our website Contact Form to get in touch with us. Or you can email a copy of the appropriate *Diet and Nutrition Worksheet(s)* and/or the appropriate *Daily Mindfulness for Life Worksheet(s)*, along with your questions and concerns. One of us will contact you as soon as possible. If you feel you have personal issues that have not been specifically addressed in this book, we encourage you to contact us. Perhaps we can offer a level of private, professional consultation and support suitable for your set of circumstances.

You may prefer to not write in the book. In that case, make copies of the worksheets or use a weekly journal to compile your thoughts. If this is your preference, we ask that you keep your record in a safe and readily accessible location where it will not be misplaced or damaged in any way. A written record of your thoughts will help you internalize what you have learned. It will also alert you to any developing or diminishing patterns of thinking or behavior that could be beneficial or hazardous to your efforts to reverse your sugar addiction.

Daily Mindfulness for Life Worksheet
(Read daily for optimal results)

1.	Was I mindful of my reactions to both pleasant and unpleasant experiences
2.	Was I able to detect sensations in my body associated with craving for sugar?
3.	Was I able to stay with a mindfulness technique for the duration of the cravings?
4.	Did I notice "feel," whether pleasant or unpleasant, in my body?
5.	What might be helpful in remembering to be mindful throughout my day?
6.	Did I feel guilty, angry or fearful, today? If so, was I aware of the mind/body components (feel, image, talk)? Did I bring a mindful awareness into the experience?
7.	How can I use mindfulness for future challenges?
8.	What are my strong points and weak points? How can mindfulness be helpful for both?
9.	Did I eat mindfully today?

Weekly Diet and Nutrition Worksheet
Week Number 1

Day of the week	Raw juices, teas, broths, or tonics drunk	Raw, cooked or steamed vegetables eaten	Raw fruits or berries eaten	Other solid food and supplements consumed
Monday				
Tuesday				
Wednesday				
Thursday				
Friday				
Saturday				
Sunday				

Comments:

Weekly Diet and Nutrition Worksheet
Week Number 2

Day of the week	Raw juices, teas, broths, or tonics drunk	Raw, cooked or steamed vegetables eaten	Raw fruits or berries eaten	Other solid food and supplements consumed
Monday				
Tuesday				
Wednesday				
Thursday				
Friday				
Saturday				
Sunday				

Comments:

Weekly Diet and Nutrition Worksheet
Week Number 3

Day of the week	Raw juices, teas, broths, or tonics drunk	Raw, cooked or steamed vegetables eaten	Raw fruits or berries eaten	Other solid food and supplements consumed
Monday				
Tuesday				
Wednesday				
Thursday				
Friday				
Saturday				
Sunday				

Comments:

Weekly Diet and Nutrition Worksheet
Week Number 4

Day of the week	Raw juices, teas, broths, or tonics drunk	Raw, cooked or steamed vegetables eaten	Raw fruits or berries eaten	Other solid food and supplements consumed
Monday				
Tuesday				
Wednesday				
Thursday				
Friday				
Saturday				
Sunday				

Comments:

Weekly Diet and Nutrition Worksheet
Week Number 5

Day of the week	Raw juices, teas, broths, or tonics drunk	Raw, cooked or steamed vegetables eaten	Raw fruits or berries eaten	Other solid food and supplements consumed
Monday				
Tuesday				
Wednesday				
Thursday				
Friday				
Saturday				
Sunday				

Comments:

BREAK OUT OF THE SUGAR PRISON

Weekly Diet and Nutrition Worksheet
Week Number 6

Day of the week	Raw juices, teas, broths, or tonics drunk	Raw, cooked or steamed vegetables eaten	Raw fruits or berries eaten	Other solid food and supplements consumed
Monday				
Tuesday				
Wednesday				
Thursday				
Friday				
Saturday				
Sunday				

Comments:

Weekly Diet and Nutrition Worksheet
Week Number 7

Day of the week	Raw juices, teas, broths, or tonics drunk	Raw, cooked or steamed vegetables eaten	Raw fruits or berries eaten	Other solid food and supplements consumed
Monday				
Tuesday				
Wednesday				
Thursday				
Friday				
Saturday				
Sunday				

Comments:

Healthy Recipes

Once you are done with the therapeutic fast or the 21-day transitional diet, you'll need to start eating nutritious meals. This is crucial if you want to help your body start the important work of rebuilding distressed organs, glands and systems.

In my experience, one of the best ways to introduce essential biochemical elements into the body is in liquid or semi-liquid form. Liquefied nutrients are easily absorbed into the bloodstream and offer the least degree of stress on the digestive organs. Over the years I have favored raw fruit and vegetable juices, health cocktails, mineral tonics, herbal teas, broths and soups to energize tired, weak and overtaxed bodies. These can rejuvenate and strengthen your body in a way that solid food cannot, regardless of nutrient density or bioavailability to the body's cells.

I am going to share with you a number of wonderful, health-promoting broths, soups, health cocktails and shakes, nut and seed milks, raw fruit juices and vegetable juice preparations. Many of which I learned from Doctor Bernard Jensen during the time I studied with him at his Hidden Valley Health Ranch, in Escondido, California.

I have added a few easy to prepare sandwiches, casseroles and other tasty, solid food recipes you should enjoy. All of which can help you reverse health issues that may have developed as a consequence of sugar and starch overindulgence.

You will notice a number of recipes calling for vegetable broth powder as seasoning. It may not be to your liking. Feel free to substitute appropriate, healthy spices for any given recipe.

Broth Recipes

Alkaline Vegetable Broth

This is the Rolls Royce of my vegetable broth formulas. This exceptionally healthy broth is one of the best simple remedies I can suggest to you for counteracting acid buildup and for many joint- and soft-tissue related pains and discomfort due to the flushing of toxic matter from your body. It is also excellent for building strength and restoring chemical balance to your body

This broth is high in organic potassium and sodium. During a healing crisis or during times of acute toxin release throughout your body, it will help to quickly neutralize your body's high acidity. If organic vegetables are not available you can use commercially grown vegetables provided they are thoroughly cleaned of surface contaminants.

Drink a cup of this alkaline broth twice daily.

4 unpeeled russet potatoes cut into half-inch squares
2 raw carrots cut into small pieces
2 sticks of raw celery cut into small pieces
6 sprigs of parsley
1/2 onion (optional)

Bring 1 quart purified water to a boil in a large pot. Add the raw vegetables, reduce heat, cover and simmer for 20 minutes. Let sit off the heat for 20 additional minutes. Drain and discard the vegetables. Refrigerate remaining broth for up to 48 hours maximum.

Vegetable Broth #2

This is easy to make. As a matter of fact, your local health food store has already done most of the work for you. Pick up a packet or small jar of organic vegetable broth powder with the primary ingredients of celery, onion, parsley, carrot and garlic. Depending on your preference, stir one or two teaspoons of the vegetable broth powder into a hot cup of organic tomato juice. Stir well and drink slowly while still warm.

Vegetable Broth #3

1 cup chopped okra
1/2 cup sweet peas
1 tablespoon vegetable broth powder (see above)
1/2 cup chopped celery, with tops
1/2 cup chopped carrots
1 medium size onion chopped fine
1 medium size white turnip chopped fine
1 cup organic tomato juice

Steam all chopped vegetables together for 10 minutes or until tender. Remove from heat. Place vegetables in a large pot. Add vegetable broth powder to taste, one pint tomato juice and one pint purified water. Add one pinch organic sea salt to enhance flavor if preferred. Reheat and serve warm.

Vegetable Broth #4

1 cup carrots
1 cup white turnips
5 strands or sprigs parsley
2 medium size white potatoes with skins
5 stalks celery with tops
1 small onion

Steam vegetables for 10 minutes or until tender. Remove from heat. Place vegetables in 1 quart purified water and add vegetable broth powder to taste. Add a pinch of organic sea salt to enhance flavor if preferred. Reheat and serve warm.

Tomato Juice and Parsley Broth

2 cups organic tomato juice
1/2 cup chopped parsley

Place parsley in a quart pot. Cover chopped parsley with cold water. Slowly bring to a boil. Remove from heat and add tomato juice. Put lid on pot and let stand for 10 minutes.

Potato and Parsley Broth

2 cups diced white potatoes
½ cup chopped parsley

Place potatoes and parsley in a quart pot. Heat one pint water on low to medium heat. Bring to a slow boil. Reduce heat and let simmer for 20 minutes. Remove from heat, stir and serve warm.

Parsley Broth

8 sprigs parsley
1 chopped small onion
1 chopped green pepper
1 teaspoon organic sweet butter
2 tablespoons vegetable broth powder
1 bunch spinach
1 chopped carrot
1 cup chopped celery with tops

Place all vegetables into pot with one quart water. Cook slowly on low to medium heat for 20 minutes. Remove from heat. Add butter, vegetable broth to taste, stir and serve warm.

Celery Broth

6 stalks chopped celery with tops
1 teaspoon organic sweet butter

Place celery in a pot with one quart water and cook slowly on low to medium heat for 20 minutes. Remove from heat. Add a small amount vegetable broth powder or sea salt to enhance flavor. Serve warm.

Onion Broth

1 large onion, finely chopped
3 diced stalks celery
1/2 cup grated cheddar cheese
1 tablespoon organic butter
2 quarts vegetable soup stock

Steam celery and onion for 10 minutes. Bring soup stock to a boil. Remove from heat. Add onion and celery and a tablespoon organic broth powder. Sprinkle with cheddar cheese.

Tomato and Celery Broth

2 cups tomato juice
1/2 cup celery juice
1 cup water

Heat tomato juice, celery juice and water on low heat for 10 minutes. Do not bring to a boil. Season with a teaspoon vegetable broth powder and a teaspoon organic butter. Serve hot.

Vegetable Broth with Rice

1 teaspoon vegetable broth powder
1/4 cup cooked brown or wild rice
1 pint water
Heat ingredients but do not boil. Serve with a teaspoon sweet organic butter or sweet cream.

Soup Recipes

Tomato Soup

4 large tomatoes
3 leeks
1 cup okra
1 medium sized onion

Finely chop leeks, okra and onion. Steam for 10 minutes. Puree tomatoes. Mix tomato puree and vegetables in 1/3 cup water. Simmer for 10 minutes. Serve with a small amount sweet cream or organic butter.

Tomato and Celery Soup

5 large tomatoes
12 stalks celery
1 quart water
1 tablespoon vegetable broth powder

Finely dice tomatoes and celery. Steam celery for 10 minutes. In a two-quart pot, add water, vegetable broth powder, tomatoes and celery. Simmer for 10 minutes, stirring periodically. Serve with organic butter to enhance flavor.

Tomato Vegetable Soup

5 large ripe tomatoes
1/2 cup chopped parsley
2 teaspoons grated onion
1 combined cup chopped celery, carrot, white potato and cabbage

Blend tomatoes with 1/4 cup water in a blender. Steam all vegetables for 15 minutes. Add all ingredients in two cups water. Heat for 10 to 15 minutes but do not bring to a boil.

Hearty Vegetable Soup

4 stalks celery
2 medium white potatoes with skins
Four medium carrots
1 small onion
1 cup chopped cabbage
2 medium tomatoes
Pinch garlic powder
2 sprigs parsley

Dice and then steam all vegetables for 10 to 15 minutes. Place in a pot with a tablespoon vegetable broth powder and one quart water. Heat until hot but not boiling. If thicker soup is desired, stir two tablespoons pure whole wheat flour into a few ounces of cold water. When the desired smoothness is obtained, add the mixture to the soup and continue heating for 5 minutes on low heat.

Celery and Parsley Soup

2 cups chopped celery tops
1 cup chopped celery stalks
1/2 cup chopped parsley
1 tablespoon vegetable broth powder

Mix all ingredients together. Cover with water and simmer for 25 minutes in a covered pot.

Green Vegetable Soup

1 cup chopped celery
1 cup chopped okra
4 stalks finely cut scallion
1 cup chopped cabbage
1 cup finely cut string beans
1 tablespoon vegetable broth powder

Combine all vegetables in a pot. Cover with water. Simmer for 25 minutes.

Down and Dirty Vegetable Soup

1/2 cup chopped cabbage
1/2 cup chopped onions
1/2 cup chopped white turnips
1/2 cup chopped white potatoes with skins
1/2 cup chopped parsnips
1/2 cup chopped carrots
6 sprigs parsley

Steam all vegetables for 10 minutes. Place in a large pot. Cover with water. Add one tablespoon vegetable broth powder or other spice. Simmer for 10 minutes.

Celery and Onion Soup

2 cups diced celery
2 medium sized chopped onions
1 tablespoon sweet butter
1 tablespoon vegetable broth powder

Place celery and onion in a pot. Cover with water. Cook on low heat for 15 minutes. Season to taste with vegetable broth powder and sweet butter.

Potato Onion Soup

4 medium diced unpeeled white potatoes
2 medium chopped onions
1 tablespoon sweet butter
1 tablespoon vegetable broth powder

Cover onions and potatoes with water. Simmer for 15 minutes. Season with vegetable broth powder and sweet butter.

Carrot and String Bean Soup

2 cups grated carrots
2 cups finely cut string beans
1 medium sized finely cut onion

Place vegetables in a pot. Cover with water, cook on low heat for 15 minutes. Season to taste with sweet butter and/or spice.

Split Pea Soup

1 cup split peas
1/2 cup sweet cream
1 small chopped onion
1/2 clove diced garlic
1 tablespoon sweet butter

Soak peas overnight in cold water. Pour water and peas into a cooking pot with onion and garlic. Be sure water just covers all ingredients. Cook on low heat until peas are mushy. Add cream and butter. Let simmer for an additional 5 minutes.

Yellow Lentil Soup

1 cup yellow lentils
1 small chopped onion
1 diced or finely cut carrot
1/2 clove diced garlic
1 tablespoon sweet butter
1 tablespoon vegetable broth powder

Soak lentils overnight in cold water. Pour water and lentils into a pot with onion, carrot, garlic and vegetable broth powder. Be sure water covers all ingredients. Cook on low heat until lentils are semi-mushy. Add butter. Let simmer for an additional 5 minutes.

Tomato Okra Soup

1 cup finely cut okra
5 large pureed tomatoes
1 pint thick almond or cashew milk
1 tablespoon vegetable broth powder
1 tablespoon sweet butter

Steam okra. Pour tomatoes, nut milk and steamed okra into a pot and simmer for 15 minutes. Season to taste with sweet butter and vegetable broth powder.

Cream of Celery Soup

1 cup finely cut celery
1 medium chopped onion

3 cups cow milk, goat milk or nut milk
2 tablespoons sweet butter
1 teaspoon vegetable broth powder

Cook celery in water for 15 minutes on low heat. Blend or stir milk, butter and vegetable broth powder together in separate container. Add mixture to celery and water. Simmer for 10 minutes.

Protein Recipes

Baked Vegetable Loaf

1 medium onion, chopped
1/2 cup finely chopped walnuts, almonds or raw peanuts
1/4 cup finely chopped celery
1/4 cup finely chopped carrots
1 well-beaten egg
1 cup whole wheat bread crumbs
2 tablespoons tomato juice
2 tablespoons melted sweet butter

Mix ingredients together and pour into a casserole dish or loaf pan. Bake for 30 minutes at 350 degrees. Serve loaf on a platter, if desired. Serve with steamed vegetables and/or raw vegetable salad.

Savory Vegetable Roast

1-1/2 cups cut asparagus
1 small onion, chopped
1 green pepper, chopped
1-1/2 cups grated cheddar cheese
1/2 teaspoon vegetable broth powder
2 eggs
1 tablespoon melted sweet butter
1 tablespoon soy flour
1/4 cup sweet cream

Blend eggs, soy flour, butter, vegetable broth powder and cream together. Pour in mixing bowl, add cheese and vegetables and mix thoroughly. Pour into a casserole dish or loaf pan and bake at 350 degrees for 35 minutes, or until done.

Baked Asparagus Loaf

1 cup hot milk
2 well-beaten eggs
4 cups asparagus, cut into one-inch pieces
3 tablespoons olive oil
1 tablespoon vegetable broth powder
1 tablespoon grated onion or onion powder
1 cup whole wheat bread crumbs
1/4 cup tomato sauce

Mix all ingredients together in casserole dish. Bake at 350 degrees for 40 minutes or until done.

Squash Loaf

1 pound summer squash
2 carrots
2 sticks celery
1 medium onion
1/2 cup whole wheat bread crumbs
2 eggs
1/2 cup milk or purified water
2 tablespoons almond butter

Shred squash, carrots, celery and onion. Place in mixing bowl. Beat almond butter, milk or water and eggs together. Add to mixing bowl and stir well. Pour into a casserole dish or loaf pan and bake at 350 degrees for 60 minutes or until done.

Lentil Roast

2 cups cooked lentils
1 medium onion, finely chopped
1 clove garlic, finely chopped

1 egg
1/2 cup milk
1 tablespoon vegetable broth powder
1/4 cup finely chopped celery

Lightly beat egg, milk and vegetable broth powder together in mixing bowl. Add lentils, onion, celery and garlic and mix together. Pour into a casserole dish or oiled loaf pan and bake at 350 degrees for 40 minutes or until done. Serve with sauce or gravy.

Lentil Patties

2 cups cooked lentils
1 well-beaten egg
1/4 cup ground raw almonds
2 tablespoons vegetable broth powder
1 teaspoon olive oil

Mash all ingredients together in a bowl or on a plate. Shape into 3-inch patties. Bake in oven on an oiled cookie sheet at 350 degrees for 30 minutes or until browned. Serve as main protein dish with sauce or gravy.

Soy Patties

2 cups cooked, mashed soybeans
1 well-beaten egg
1 small onion, finely chopped
1/3 cup whole wheat bread crumbs
1/2 teaspoon vegetable broth powder

Mash all ingredients together in a bowl or on a plate. Shape into 3-inch patties. Bake in oven on an oiled cookie sheet at 350 degrees for 30 minutes or until browned. Serve as main protein dish with sauce or gravy.

Soy and Lentil Loaf

1 cup cooked lentil puree
2 cups cooked soybean puree
5 tablespoons sweet cream
1 medium onion, grated
1/2 teaspoon sage or basil
1 tablespoon olive oil

Mix ingredients together. Pour into a casserole dish or loaf pan. Bake at 350 degrees for 50 minutes. Serve as main protein dish with sauce or gravy.

Lentil Loaf

2 cups cooked lentils
1 well-beaten egg
1 cup whole wheat bread crumbs
1 cup diced celery
1 tablespoon finely minced onion
1 teaspoon vegetable broth powder
1/2 cup tomato paste

Mix together in a bowl. Pour into a casserole dish or loaf pan and bake at 350 degrees for 25 minutes or until done.

Soy Loaf

1 cup cooked brown rice
1 cup cooked soybeans
1/2 cup tomato juice

1 cup whole wheat bread crumbs
1 tablespoon minced onion
1 teaspoon vegetable broth powder
1 tablespoon olive oil
1 heaping tablespoon soy flour
1 well-beaten egg

Mix all ingredients together in mixing bowl. Pour into a casserole dish or loaf pan and bake at 350 degrees for 30 minutes or until done.

Soya Casserole

2 cups cooked, mashed soybeans
1 cup whole wheat bread crumbs
1 cup grated carrots
1/2 cup finely chopped celery
1 well-beaten egg
1 medium onion, finely chopped
1 clove garlic, finely chopped
2 cups milk
2 teaspoons vegetable broth powder

Combine all ingredients in a bowl and mix thoroughly. Pour into a casserole dish, cover and bake at 350 degrees for 90 minutes or until done.

Soy and Egg Loaf

1/2 pound cooked, mashed soybeans
2 well-beaten eggs
2 tablespoons chopped parsley
1/2 cup finely chopped celery
1 small onion, finely chopped
2 teaspoons vegetable broth powder

Mix all ingredients together in a bowl. Pour into a casserole dish or loaf pan and bake at 350 degrees for 25 minutes.

Soy and Vegetable Loaf

3 cups cooked, mashed soybeans
1 small onion, finely chopped
1/4 cup finely chopped celery
1/2 cup cooked tomatoes
1/2 cup finely chopped green peppers
1 tablespoon olive oil

Mix ingredients together in a bowl. Pour into a casserole dish or loaf pan and bake at 350 degrees for 50 minutes. Serve with sauce or gravy.

Vegetarian Soy Loaf

2 cups cooked soybeans
1/2 cup finely chopped green peppers
1 medium onion, finely chopped
1/4 cup chopped parsley
1 cup finely chopped celery
1 cup cooked tomatoes
1 teaspoon vegetable broth powder

Mix ingredients together. Pour into a casserole dish or loaf pan and bake at 350 degrees for 35 minutes or until tender. Serve with sauce or gravy.

Healthy Nut Roast

1 cup grated carrots
1 small onion, finely chopped

3 tablespoons raw almond or cashew butter
1 cup milk
1 cup finely chopped celery
1/2 cup whole wheat bread crumbs
1 egg

Blend egg, milk and nut butter together. Mix together with all other ingredients in a bowl. Bake in casserole dish at 350 degrees for 50 minutes. Serve with sauce or gravy.

Carrot Pecan Loaf

2 cups grated carrots
1/2 cup finely cut raw pecans
1/2 cup milk
1 small onion, finely chopped
1/2 cup whole wheat bread crumbs
1 egg

Blend egg and milk together. Mix together with all other ingredients in a bowl. Bake in oven at 350 degrees for 70 minutes or until done. Serve with sauce or gravy.

Walnut Lentil Loaf

1 cup cooked lentils
1 cup finely chopped raw walnuts
1/2 cup chopped celery
1 small onion, finely chopped
1 egg
1/2 cup milk
1 teaspoon vegetable broth powder

Blend egg and milk together. Mix lightly together with all other ingredients in a bowl. Bake in casserole dish at 350 degrees for 50 minutes. Serve with sauce or gravy.

Holiday Season Apple Celery Nut Roast

1-1/2 cups finely chopped celery with tops
1/2 cup finely chopped raw almonds
1 cup chopped apples
1 cup whole wheat bread crumbs
1 egg
1 cup milk

Blend egg and milk together. Mix together with all other ingredients. Bake in casserole dish at 350 degrees for 45 minutes.

Thanksgiving Walnut Loaf

1 cup grated carrots
1 cup finely chopped raw walnuts
1 cup whole wheat bread crumbs
1 cup chopped, strained tomatoes
1-1/2 tablespoons melted sweet butter
4 well-beaten eggs
1 teaspoon vegetable broth powder

Mix all ingredients together in a bowl. Bake in a casserole dish at 350 degrees for 60 minutes. Serve plain or with gravy.

Baked and Cooked Vegetables

Steamed Onions and Tomatoes

1 bell pepper coarsely cut
2 cups finely chopped tomatoes
1 cup diced onions
1 teaspoon vegetable broth powder
1 tablespoon melted sweet butter
2 tablespoons grated cheddar cheese
2 sprigs parsley

Mix vegetables, butter and vegetable broth powder together. Steam until onions are tender. Cover with cheese and parsley sprigs and serve.

Eggplant Okra Casserole

2 cups cooked diced eggplant
1 cup cooked okra
3/4 cup sliced tomatoes
1 tablespoon melted sweet butter
1/2 cup whole wheat bread crumbs
1 teaspoon vegetable broth powder

Alternate okra, eggplant and tomatoes in layers in casserole dish. Sprinkle vegetable broth powder over each successive layer. Cover with bread crumbs and sweet butter. Bake at 350 degrees for 50 minutes. Serve with mushroom sauce.

Baked Vegetable Medley

4 medium-sized new potatoes
3 carrots

5 small white onions
3 small red beets
1 rutabaga
1 tablespoon melted sweet butter

Cut carrots and potatoes once lengthwise. Slice beets and rutabaga into eighths. Leave onions whole. Place in casserole dish with enough water to cover bottom. Bake at 350 degrees for 20 minutes or until vegetables are thoroughly cooked and tender, but not wilted. Add sweet butter and serve.

Vegetable Chop Suey

1 cup dried mushrooms
1 cup chopped celery
2 cups bean sprouts
2 large onions, chopped
1/2 cup water chestnuts
1/4 cup raw walnuts

Soak mushrooms for 4 hours in a large bowl. Use enough water to cover mushrooms entirely. Add all other ingredients and add enough extra water to cover all ingredients. Simmer on stove until all vegetables are tender. Separate vegetables and nuts from remaining water and serve with cooked brown rice, soy sauce, sweet and sour sauce, or any other appropriate and tasty spices desired. Note: You can use fresh mushrooms instead and simply simmer them with the other ingredients.

Vegetable Stew

3 white turnips cut into ½-inch cubes
2 carrots cut into ½-inch lengths
4 medium onions cut into eight sections
4 sticks celery cut into ½-inch lengths

1 bay leaf
1/2 clove garlic
2 tablespoons whole wheat flour
1/2 pound tofu or other soy-based meat substitute cut into small sections
3 medium tomatoes, quartered
1 tablespoon melted sweet butter
1/2 teaspoon celery salt or vegetable broth powder

Use enough water to cover turnips, carrots, onions, celery, bay leaf and garlic completely. Simmer for 20 minutes. Add tofu or meat substitute, tomatoes and seasoning. Mix flour separately with enough cold water to make a smooth paste. Add the paste to the other ingredients and simmer for 10 minutes or until thickened. Add butter and serve.

Baked Onions and Tomatoes

1 bell pepper coarsely cut
2 cups chopped tomatoes (coarsely cut if preferred)
1 medium onion, diced
1/4 cup chopped parsley
1 tablespoon melted sweet butter
2 tablespoons grated cheddar cheese
1 teaspoon vegetable broth powder

Mix vegetables, butter and seasoning together. Pour into casserole dish. Cover with grated cheese and bake at 350 degrees for 30 minutes. Garnish with cut parsley sprigs and serve.

Baked Stuffed Zucchini

2 pounds zucchini
1 large bell pepper
3 tablespoons chopped parsley

1 teaspoon vegetable broth powder
1/2 cup grated Parmesan cheese
1/2 cup tomato juice

Cut each zucchini lengthwise and scoop out inside. Place zucchini boats inside a large flat casserole dish or other baking dish or pan. Mix scooped out portions with all other ingredients. Place mixture inside zucchini sections and cover with tomato juice. Bake at 350 degrees for 20 minutes.

Hippocrates Vegetable Casserole

4 medium white potatoes
1 medium onion
2 carrots
1 small bell pepper
5 medium mushrooms
2 tablespoons olive oil
1 teaspoon pure lemon juice

Cut all vegetables into one-or half-inch pieces. Place in a large bowl. Add olive oil and lemon juice. Add a pinch of sea salt if desired. Mix together thoroughly by hand. Pour all ingredients into a large casserole dish. Bake at 350 degrees for 50 minutes or until done.

Sandwiches

You can use most whole grain and sprouted breads for these sandwich combinations. It is always best to have the bread unheated, however, light toasting is permitted. (Whole grain rye and sprouted wheat are two of my favorites.) Try a few of these little-known healthy sandwich combinations. You will be surprised at how satisfying they can be to your stomach and palate. For a sandwich spread, try something other than mayonnaise. Your local health store has plenty of healthy and tasty variations to choose from. Please note that any recipe calling for honey may possibly trigger honey bingeing.

- Avocado sliced or mashed with romaine lettuce.
- Avocado sliced or mashed with alfalfa sprouts.
- Lettuce, grated carrots, raisins and cream cheese.
- Dates, nuts and cream cheese.
- Figs and cream cheese.
- Lettuce, grated celery and grated carrots with Swiss cheese.
- Nut butter, olives and sliced watercress.
- Banana slices, cashew butter, honey.
- Banana slices, almond butter and grated coconut.
- Sliced cucumber and cream cheese.
- Swiss cheese, sliced cucumber, alfalfa sprouts.
- Cottage cheese and green onion.
- Cottage cheese and strawberry slices.
- Cream cheese, thin pineapple slices and thin apple slices
- Cottage cheese and walnut or pecans.

- Cottage cheese and slices of watercress.
- Cream cheese, nuts and raisins.
- Raisins, dates, figs, nuts and cream cheese.
- Apple sauce mixed half and half with almond or cashew butter.
- Pecan or cashew butter mixed half and half with chopped, pitted olives.
- Cream cheese, almond butter and lettuce.

Fruit and Vegetable Cocktails

Each of the following blended cocktail combinations can help deliver important nutrients to your cells. These can be consumed with or between meals. Please note that predominantly or exclusively fruit drinks should not be combined with starchy vegetable or grain-product foods. Predominantly or exclusively vegetable cocktails should not be consumed at the same meal where acid and sub-acid fruits are eaten. Some of the following combinations can trigger strong cleansing reactions which are beneficial, but often unpleasant. If this is the case, either stop drinking a particular beverage or dilute it with purified water until you no longer experience any unpleasant reactions. Please note that any recipe calling for honey may possibly trigger honey bingeing.

Blood and body builders:

- 1/2 coconut milk, 1/2 fig juice.
- 1/2 coconut milk and 1/2 carrot juice.
- 1/2 carrot juice and 1/2 whole, raw goat milk.
- 1/4 red beet and leaf juice, one cucumber, 1/4 celery juice and 1/4 pineapple juice.
- 1/4 red beet juice, 1/4 white turnip juice, 1/4 celery juice and 1/4 carrot juice.
- 1/4 spinach juice, 1/4 parsley juice, 1/4 carrot juice and 1/4 cucumber juice.
- 1/2 celery juice, 1/4 carrot juice, 1/8 spinach juice and 1/8 parsley juice.

For my personal, body building and blood mineralizing nutritional formula I drink at least four days every week, check my Whole Foods Blended Cocktail recipe described on page 157 of the Appendix.

Vitality and energy tonics:

- 1/3 celery juice and 2/3 orange juice.
- 1/2 celery juice, 1/4 pineapple juice and 1/4 apple juice.
- 1/2 orange juice, 1/2 pomegranate juice and a teaspoon of raw honey.
- 1/3 pineapple juice, 1/3 apple juice, 1/3 grapefruit juice and a pinch of lemon juice. (This is an excellent high sodium drink to help keep you cool in hot weather).
- 1/4 apple juice, 1/4 pineapple juice, 1/4 celery juice and 1/4 strawberry juice.
- 1/2 cabbage juice, 1/2 pineapple juice and a tablespoon of raw almonds butter.
- 1/2 celery juice, 1/4 carrot juice and 1/4 parsley juice.
- 1/3 white turnip juice, 1/3 celery juice, 1/3 parsley juice and a pinch of radish juice.
- 1/4 pineapple juice, quarter strawberry juice, 1/4 celery juice and 1/4 orange juice. (This is another cooling drink due to the high concentration of organic sodium).

Skin, nails and hair care:

- 1/2 oat straw tea, 1/4 celery juice, 1/4 fig juice and a pinch of dulse or kelp.
- 1/3 cucumber juice, 1/3 parsley juice and 1/3 pineapple juice.
- Mix equal parts of cucumber juice, watercress juice, celery juice, tomato juice, cucumber juice and parsley juice.

- Mix equal parts of oat straw tea, spinach juice, parsley juice, pineapple juice and celery juice.
- Mix equal parts of strawberry juice, rhubarb juice, pineapple juice and celery juice.

Nut and Seed Milks

Nut and seed milks are a wonderful way to supply essential minerals and high-quality proteins to your body. There are specific formulas that can be much more nutritious and healthy for you than cow milk or other dairy products. Many preparations can be used as suitable and nutritious substitutes for cow milk for infants. When I prepare a nut or seed milk, I throw everything into a blender and set it on high for 2 minutes. If I am looking for a milky consistency, I finely strain the blended mixture. Sometimes I like to drink the entire blended formula, especially if I have added a number of whole food extracts or supplements to the mixture before blending. Experiment so you can determine what works best for you. Please note that any recipe calling for honey may possibly trigger honey bingeing.

Following is the specific nut and seed milk recipe mentioned in the protocol for this book.

Nut and Seed Milk Recipe for the Protocol

This alkalinizing nut and seed milk - high in protein, calcium and other essential nutrients – is helpful for systemic acidity, circulatory and heart related complications, and irregularity. It can also be beneficial in cases of sugar fermentation due to systemic carbonosis.

Place the following ingredients into a blender:

¼ cup raw almonds (dry or previously soaked overnight in water or pineapple juice)
1 tablespoon raw, hulled, sesame seeds or raw tahini
1 tablespoon raw sunflower seeds
1 tablespoon raw flaxseeds
1 quart purified water and 3 ice cubes
1 tablespoon cold pressed, organic safflower or sunflower oil

Blend together for approximately 2 minutes. Strain the mixture through cheese cloth or use a metal strainer, pressing down the mixture with a spoon or spatula. Use immediately or store in refrigerator until ready for use. Shake well before using. It will stay fresh in refrigerator for 3 days.

Drink this nut and seed milk 3 or 4 days out of each week, preferably at lunch or as a between meals snack. It is excellent as a healthy substitute for cow milk. When I make this nut and seed milk, I do not use anything as a sweetener.

Other Tasty Nut and Seed Milks

- 3 tablespoons coconut milk, one cup pineapple juice, one cup water.
- 3 tablespoons tahini butter (sesame seeds), one teaspoon raw honey and 12 ounces purified water.
- 2 tablespoons almond butter or 1/4 cup raw almonds, one teaspoon raw honey and one pint purified water.
- 2 tablespoons almond butter, one tablespoon tahini, one cup orange juice and 1/2 cup purified water.
- 1 tablespoon tahini, 1/4 cup raw sunflower seeds, 1 tablespoon almond butter, 1 teaspoon raw honey and 12 ounces purified water.
- 2 tablespoons coconut milk, 1 tablespoon tahini, 1 tablespoon almond butter and a teaspoon honey.
- 1/2 cup brown rice or a brown and wild rice mixture, 1/4 cup raw oats, 1 tablespoon raw eucalyptus honey or rice bran syrup, 1 quart purified water. Blend ingredients together for two minutes, strain and refrigerate. Use within 72 hours. This is a grain milk recipe that is strengthening to the muscular system, beneficial to the entire endocrine system and excellent in helping keep blood vessel walls soft and pliable. It is a wonderful tonic for the cerebellum as well, being high in potassium and silicon.

Raw Vegetable Salads

Healthy, interesting and tasty raw vegetable salads can be constructed in numerous ways from the following list of vegetables. As you discover other vegetables not included on the list, add them to your diet and be sure to try them periodically.

- Asparagus
- Beets
- Beet greens
- Broccoli
- Brussels sprouts
- Cabbage
- Carrot
- Cauliflower
- Celery
- Celery tops
- Corn
- Cucumber
- Dandelion greens
- Egg plant
- Endive
- Kohlrabi
- Leeks
- Lettuce - butter, red leaf and romaine
- Mushrooms
- Okra
- Olives
- Onion
- Peas
- Radishes
- Rhubarb

- Sea weed
- Sorrel
- Spinach
- Sprouts - particularly alfalfa
- String beans
- Swiss chard
- Tomato
- Turnips
- Watercress

This wraps up our special recipes section. Hopefully you will return here often to try many, if not all, of the tasty, healthy foods and beverages. Immediately following are two especially healthy recipes. I often use these in my clinical work with patients. Perhaps you will find them to be helpful on the road to whole-being health and wellness.

Silicon Tonic Recipe

This is one of the best natural stimulants for the cerebellum — your body's electrical battery and overseer of sexual and muscular activity. Regardless of what your blood sugar level may be, when the cerebellum is underperforming, you will feel tired, irritable, despondent and enervated. If you will try this marvelous elixir, along with the dietary suggested in this book, within a short time you should notice a resurgence of energy, sexual interest and muscular strength.

I recommend that you add this wonderful brain and nerve tonic to your daily menu as soon as you finish the therapeutic fast or the 21-day transitional diet.

Put 1 tablespoon each of whole barley, whole oats and raw wheat bran in a pint of purified water. Shake briskly and refrigerate for at least eight hours. Strain the water, throw away the bulk, heat the water on your stove until it is warm - not boiling - and slowly drink 1 cup. You can also let the strained tonic sit in sunlight for an hour before drinking — which is my preferred method. Refrigerate what's left. It'll be good for one more day.

I have found that the addition of a tablespoon of liquid chlorophyll to this tonic gives a noticeable boost in energy as the day unfolds.

Whole Foods Blended Cocktail – Energizing and Body Building Drink

Mix the following ingredients with 8 to 10 ounces of purified water and blend together until smooth. Drink *slowly* during breakfast or lunch or as a healthy snack.

- Brown rice protein powder or whey protein powder – 15 grams
- Raw flaxseeds – 1 tablespoon
- Raw bee pollen – 1 teaspoon, or a serving of royal jelly (**Caution:** DO NOT use bee pollen or royal jelly if you are allergic to either)
- Wheat germ oil – 1 teaspoon
- Kelp – 3 tablets or ½ teaspoon of powder or granules
- Chlorella - 10 tablets of 200 milligram size. May cause gas initially
- Brewer's yeast – 2 tablespoons. May cause gas initially
- Lecithin – one tablespoon or follow directions on container for a single serving
- Full spectrum vitamin preparation – made from whole foods.
- Natural digestive aid for protein, fats and carbohydrates – find one that has HCL and pepsin or (preferably) use one half tablespoon of organic apple cider vinegar as a substitute
- Multi-mineral supplement with chromium and manganese – both trace minerals assist in the control and efficient metabolism of sugar

This is an excellent energizing and body-building cocktail that can help restore structural integrity of your body's systems and assist with restoring efficient function of same. I have taken this cocktail, or a similar preparation, at least 4 mornings out of every week, for the past 2 decades, to great advantage. What I have discovered, to my delight, is that soon after drinking this healthy cocktail on an empty stomach or with very little solid food (such as a tablespoon of raw wheat germ), my body and mind enjoy a steady flow of subtle, sustained energy for, at least, 5 hours.

References

Articles

Davidson, R.J., Kabat-Zinn, J. Schumacher, J., Rosenkranz, M., Miller, D., Santorelli, S.F., Urbanowski, F., Harrington, A., Bonus, K., Sheridan, J.F. (2003) Alteration in brain and immune function produced by mindfulness meditation, *Psychosomatic Medicine*, 65, 564-570.

Creswell, D., (UCLA) (2007), Brain scans reveal why meditation works, *Psychosomatic Medicine*

Baer, R., (2006), Mindfulness-based approaches to eating disorders, New York: Guilford Press, 76-91

Kristeller, J.L., Hallett, B. (1999), Effects of meditation-based intervention in the treatment of binge eating. *Journal of Health Psychology*. 4(3) 357-363

Stein, J. (2003), The one-minute meditator: connecting with inner wisdom. *Time*

Plesman, J., (2005), The Connection Between Depression, Addiction, and Hypoglycemia?
The Hypoglycemic Association of Australia

Henkel, J., (2006) Sugar Substitutes: Americans Opt for Sweetness and Lite.
Sugar in the morning, sugar in the evening, sugar at suppertime.
FDA Consumer

USDA, Economic Research Service Bulletin Number 33

Rosen, S., Shapoiri, S., (2008), Obesity in the Midst of Unyielding Food Insecurity in Developing Countries U.S.D.A., *Amber Waves*

Cheraskin, E., (2003), The Ideal Blood Sugar. *Wise Traditions in Food, Farming and the Healing Arts*

News Story

Victory, J., (2006), *"Studying The Sweet Tooth," ABC NEWS*

Books

Young, S., (2004), *Break Through Pain: A Step by Step Mindfulness Meditation Program for Transforming Chronic and Acute Pain*

Hopkins, J., Lama, Dalai, *How To Practice: The Way To A Meaningful Life*

Nebelsieck, A., Rinpoche, Z., *The Backdoor To Enlightenment*

Mindfulness-Based Approaches To Eating Disorders, Guilford Press

Taber, C. W., *Taber's Cyclopedic Medical Dictionary*, Ninth Edition

Jensen, B., *Vibrant Health from Your Kitchen*

Jensen, B., *Beyond Basic Health – Advanced Thinking For The Healing Arts*

Esser, W., *Dictionary of Natural Foods*

Lindlahr, H., *Iridiagnosis and Other Diagnostic Methods*, Volume IV – Natural Therapeutics

REFERENCES

Vogel, A., *Swiss Nature Doctor*

Walker, N., *Fresh Vegetable and Fruit Juices*

Christopher, J., *School of Natural Healing*

Lust, John B., *The Herb Book*

Waerland, A., *The Cauldron of Disease*

Airola, P., *How to Get Well*

Thayer, G., *Health for One Hundred Years*

Shelton, H., *The Science and Fine Art of Food and Nutrition*

Jensen, B., M. Anderson., *Empty Harvest*

Rothenberg, R., *Medical Dictionary and Health Manual*

Chapman, J., Perry, E., *The Biochemic Handbook - Biochemic Theory and Practice*

Gray, H., *Gray's Anatomy: The Classic Collector's Edition*

Mindfulness Daily Practice Flash Cards

On the following pages there are 20 mindfulness daily practice flash cards. Cut out or, preferably, make copies of the flash cards. Then cut out the copies and keep at least one flash card with you throughout each day of the entire protocol. Research has proven that flash cards with relevant inspirational affirmations have been effective in helping to reverse addictive tendencies. Keep one in your pocket book, purse, wallet or in a pant, shirt, blouse or coat pocket. When you feel the urge to binge on some form of sugar or sugar byproduct, or to discontinue the protocol we recommend in the book, pull out the card and read it silently or aloud.

I will not eat refined sugar today.	I will stay present with what arises both within myself and outside myself.
I will stay with my technique until the urge has passed or it no longer has power over me.	I am strong enough to get through a craving without acting on it.
I will live through the pain of deprivation and be so happy when I come out the other side.	I NEVER regret abstinence. I AWAYS regret binging.

I am not perfect and this is perfect.	Today I will maintain loving kindness towards myself and others.
I can get through any craving for sugar without acting on it.	I will practice sitting meditation and meditation in action today.
If I am upset, I will IMMEDIATELY, without hesitation, apply a mindfulness technique.	I will walk through my resistances just for today.

MINDFULNESS DAILY PRACTICE FLASH CARDS

I will allow nature to cleanse, purify, strengthen and rebuild my body from inside out.	The better I feed my body, the stronger it will be and the better it will perform.
I will eat and drink only those foods and beverages that can help restore a healthy body.	The sugar I sought from candy, cakes, pies and soft drinks were harmful. What I need for my body can be supplied by whole, nutritious foods and beverages and natural food supplements.
I will complete the seven day fast to cleanse, rest and strengthen my body.	I will complete the 21-day transitional diet to cleanse, rest and strengthen my body.

I will follow the daily maintenance menu I have chosen to help build healthy, strong tissue in my body.	I will not abuse my body anymore by bingeing on sugar, starchy foods or fatty foods.

To Contact the Authors

Shelly Young, MA, LPC, CAC III
Email: shelly@breakoutofthesugarprison.com
URL: http://www.breakoutofthesugarprison.com

Paul Harris, BS, CN, CI
Email: paul@breakoutofthesugarprison.com
URL: http://www.breakoutofthesugarprison.com

About the Authors

Shelly Young, MA, LPC, CAC III, is a licensed professional counselor and certified addiction counselor. She has been a mindfulness instructor for over 25 years and has led workshops and trainings throughout the U.S. and Canada since 1985.

Shelly has led mindfulness trainings at the University of Colorado Health Sciences Center, Sierra Tucson Treatment Center, University of New Mexico, JFK University, Longmont United Hospital, Denver Health Addiction Counselor Training Program, and many other health education facilities. She has presented Grand Rounds lectures at numerous hospitals including Bethesda Naval Medical Center.

Shelly's course, *Mindfulness: a Treatment Approach for Addictive Compulsive Behavior* was approved by the Alcohol and Drug Abuse Division of the State of Colorado as an elective for addiction counselor trainees. She has led continuing education seminars for mental health and medical professionals in over 100 U.S. cities. Presently she maintains a private practice near Boulder, Colorado. Her focus is on mindfulness-based psychotherapy and pain management.

Today Shelly is free from what was once a devastating sugar and food addiction.

Paul Harris, BS, CN, CI, is a certified nutritionist who has been practicing complementary alternative medicine since 1985.

The health-restoring biological therapies and natural healing methodologies he teaches and administers to patients were largely inspired by world-renowned natural health care advocate, lecturer, author and practitioner, Bernard Jensen, DC, ND, PhD. He studied under Dr. Jensen from 1984 until 1995 at Hidden Valley Health Ranch in Escondido, California. Paul spent 21 years as a practice development and physician recruitment consultant to allopathic and osteopathic medical groups and hospital management. It was during this time that he gained a clear understanding of the many forces and mindsets controlling America's health care industry.

Paul currently consults with clients, visitors to his websites and with readers of his publications. He enjoys helping people find and unfold their unique potential through healthy and productive living.

Made in the USA
Lexington, KY
05 February 2011